Essentials in Ophthalmology

Series Editor

Arun D. Singh, Cleveland Clinic Foundation
Cole Eye Institute, Cleveland, OH, USA

Essentials in Ophthalmology aims to promote the rapid and efficient transfer of medical research into clinical practice. It is published in four volumes per year. Covering new developments and innovations in all fields of clinical ophthalmology, it provides the clinician with a review and summary of recent research and its implications for clinical practice. Each volume is focused on a clinically relevant topic and explains how research results impact diagnostics, treatment options and procedures as well as patient management.

The reader-friendly volumes are highly structured with core messages, summaries, tables, diagrams and illustrations and are written by internationally well-known experts in the field. A volume editor supervises the authors in his/her field of expertise in order to ensure that each volume provides cutting-edge information most relevant and useful for clinical ophthalmologists. Contributions to the series are peer reviewed by an editorial board.

Vishal R. Raval • Prithvi Mruthyunjaya
Arun D. Singh
Editors

Ocular and Adnexal Lymphoma

Second Edition

Springer

Editors
Vishal R. Raval
Anant Bajaj Retina Institute
The Operation Eyesight Universal
Institute for Eye Cancer
L V Prasad Eye Institute
Hyderabad, Telangana, India

Prithvi Mruthyunjaya
Stanford Medicine
Palo Alto, CA, USA

Arun D. Singh
Cleveland Clinic
Cole Eye Institute
Cleveland, OH, USA

ISSN 1612-3212 ISSN 2196-890X (electronic)
Essentials in Ophthalmology
ISBN 978-3-031-24594-7 ISBN 978-3-031-24595-4 (eBook)
https://doi.org/10.1007/978-3-031-24595-4

This Springer imprint is published by the registered company Springer Nature Switzerland AG
The registered company address is: Gewerbestrasse 11, 6330 Cham, Switzerland

Preface

Ocular and adnexal lymphomas are rare and diverse; hence their diagnosis and treatment usually require special expertise. Increasingly, the care of such a patient is provided by a multidisciplinary team comprising ocular oncologists, general oncologists, pathologists, radiation oncologists, and other specialists. The field of lymphoma is advancing rapidly because of accelerating progress in tumor biology, pharmacology, and the advent of targeted therapies. For all these reasons, we felt that there was scope for a new edition of the monograph regarding ocular and adnexal lymphoma.

To harmonize the terminology across this monograph the editors have taken the liberty of labeling vitreo-retinal lymphoma as PCNSL-O as the preferred term to emphasize that it is an ocular variant or subset of primary CNS lymphoma (PCNSL). Those with concurrent CNS and ocular disease may be labeled as PCNSL-CNS/O in contrast to patients with CNS only involvement (PCNSL-CNS) at presentation. This monograph, a conjoint effort of ocular oncologists, general oncologists, and pathologists, comprises 11 chapters covering molecular pathology, clinical features, and treatment. It is our sincere hope that this monograph will provide a useful resource for providing appropriate care to our patients.

Hyderabad, Telangana, India — Vishal R. Raval
Palo Alto, CA, USA — Prithvi Mruthyunjaya
Cleveland, OH, USA — Arun D. Singh

Acknowledgments

This, my first book, would not have taken shape without the guidance of my mentor, Dr. Arun D Singh, Director of Ophthalmic Oncology, Cole Eye Institute, Cleveland Clinic, Ohio, USA. My deep and sincere gratitude to Dr. Singh for the opportunity, and for the privilege and honor to have worked and studied under him.

I must thank the Hyderabad Eye Research Institute, Hyderabad, for their support and contribution throughout my research career.

I am also grateful to my parents for their love, prayers, care, and their many sacrifices to support my education and career. I can always count on my wife, Shaily, and my daughters, Drishti and Deeti, for their love, understanding, faith, and steady support throughout my research career (Vishal).

To my parents who educated me beyond their means, my wife, Annapurna, and my children, Nakul and Rahul, who make all my efforts worthwhile (Arun Singh).

For all I have learned from the pearls of my mentors and the journey of my patients. Grateful to my late father who taught me the value of helping those in need (Prithivi).

Contents

1 Primary Central Nervous System Lymphoma: Terminology and Outcome Measures

Arun D. Singh and Vishal R. Raval

Introduction

Central nervous system (CNS) is rarely affected by lymphoma, either as a primary site or as secondary site with prior non-CNS involvement [1]. In either case, diffuse large B cell lymphoma (DLBCL) is the most frequent variant [2]. Other less common subtypes include Burkitt lymphoma, mantle cell lymphoma, and anaplastic large cell lymphoma [3]. Histologic subtypes of lymphoma that most frequently affect ocular adnexa such as extranodal marginal zone lymphoma, follicular lymphoma, lymphoplasmacytic lymphoma, and chronic lymphocytic leukemia/small lymphocytic lymphoma rarely affect the CNS [3].

Terminology

To a large extent, vitreoretinal lymphoma mimics the pattern of CNS lymphoma. However, there is a lack of consensus regarding appropriate terminology for primary CNS lymphoma (PCNSL) involving the ocular compartment. Historically CNS lymphoma involving the eye was described as reticulum cell sarcoma [4] and microgliomatosis [5]. In the last two decades, terminology such as intraocular lymphoma (IOL) has been introduced [6]. However, this term is confusing as it does not differentiate lymphoma involving such as the retina and vitreous (high grade DLBCL subtype) from lymphoma involving the uveal tract (low grade extranodal marginal zone lymphoma) [7]. Vitreoretinal lymphoma (VRL) is the most commonly used term in the literature; however, it implies that the disease originates in the eye [8].

We suggest PCNSL-O as the preferred term to emphasize that it is an ocular variant or subset of PCNSL [9, 10]. Those with concurrent CNS and ocular disease may be labeled as (PCNSL-CNS/O) in contrast to patients with CNS only involvement (PCNSL-CNS) at presentation.

PCNSL is a subtype of non-Hodgkin lymphoma confined to the CNS compartments. As per the 2017 World Health Organization classification of hematopoietic and lymphoid tumors [11], PCNSL is classified as primary DLBCL of the CNS. The CNS compartments include the brain (deep cortical regions, periventricular regions, and basal ganglia), spinal cord, meninges, and eyes [12]. The involvement of the eye and other CNS compartments varies as ophthalmic manifestations can precede, occur simultaneously with or follow disease in other CNS sites.

A. D. Singh (✉)
Cole Eye Institute, Cleveland Clinic, Cleveland, OH, USA
e-mail: singha@ccf.org

V. R. Raval
Anant Bajaj Retina Institute, The Operation Eyesight Universal Institute for Eye Cancer, L V Prasad Eye Institute, Hyderabad, Telangana, India

V. R. Raval et al. (eds.), *Ocular and Adnexal Lymphoma*, Essentials in Ophthalmology,
https://doi.org/10.1007/978-3-031-24595-4_1

Sixty percent to 90% of patients with ocular involvement ultimately involve other CNS compartments, while 20% of patients with PCNSL present with concurrent ocular involvement [13, 14]. The median interval between the progression of lymphoma from the eye to other CNS compartments and vice versa varies over a follow-up of 8–29 months [12, 13, 15]. The overall prognosis of ocular involved PCNSL is also poor, because of CNS involvement with 5-year survival rates between 25% and 40% [16].

Secondary vitreoretinal lymphoma also follows pattern similar to that of secondary CNS lymphoma with DLBCL being the predominant lymphoma subtypes identified by retinal biopsy [17, 18]. Uncommon vitreoretinal involvement in the setting of cutaneous peripheral T-cell lymphoma, the NK-T cell lymphoma and adult T-cell lymphoma/leukemia and CNS T-cell lymphoma has also been reported [19–23].

Outcomes

Currently, the management of PCNSL-O is focused on local ocular control, given insufficient evidence that ocular treatment decreases progression to CNS [10, 24]. Despite achieving high rates of local ocular control with intravitreal agents including methotrexate [25] and rituximab [10, 26].

Additional secondary and tertiary outcome measures of progression-free survival (PFS) and overall survival (OS), respectively, should also be reported.

Primary Outcome

Assessment of local treatment response in the eye and CNS compartments is the primary outcome measure. Local treatment response can be assessed using terminology and criteria proposed by International PCNSL Collaborative Group for standardization of baseline evaluation and response criteria for primary CNS lymphoma [27].

- Complete response (CR); no evidence of residual disease within the anterior eye chamber, vitreous cavity, or retina
- Partial response (PR): 50% or greater reduction in ocular disease
- Progressive disease (PD): 25% increase of ocular manifestations compared to pretreatment assessment

Two additional concepts specific to PCNSL-O need special mention

- Relapse in local ocular disease or recurrence after a defined period of CR. This is not synonymous as progression of lymphoma into CNS compartment and it is preferable not to include such cases with compartmental progression for reporting of progression-free survival (PFS)
- Minimal residual disease (MRD) concept of subclinical tumor burden is used frequently in the management of leukemias [28]. A similar concept of MRD in treatment and staging of vitreoretinal lymphoma is recommended [29] as most of the patients at the end of treatment are left with residual vitreous opacities/debris which seems to be clinically nonactive. However, without sure knowledge of the origin of those opacities, it is not entirely correct to label such a patient as a complete response (CR). Therefore, at minimum ophthalmologists should document the presence or absence of all vitreous opacities using a graded scale.

Secondary Outcome: Progression-Free Survival (PFS)

Given that PCNSL-O is a subset of PCNSL [9] with a strong propensity to progress to the CNS, treatment effectiveness should not be evaluated solely in terms of local ocular response [10]. Most retrospective studies have defined PFS as time from onset of symptoms [30] or diagnosis to progression or relapse/death [31–34]. PFS defined in this way results in heterogeneous outcomes such as local relapse, progression, and death making results among studies non-comparable. The lack of well-defined outcome measures, particularly related to progression, further hampers valid comparisons between published studies [10].

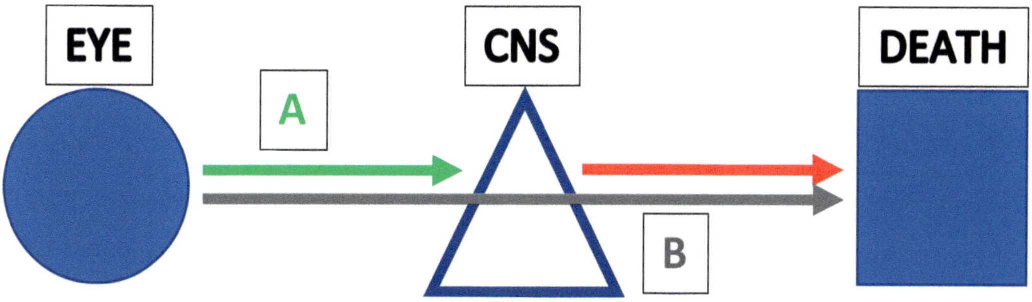

Fig. 1.1 Schematic representation of intercompartmental progression of a patient with PCNSL-O from presentation to death. The PFS is represented by a green arrow (interval A) and red arrow (interval B) for patients with PCNSL-O. The gray arrow (interval B) represents OS for a patient with PCNSL-O. Representation of PFS as intercompartmental progression is important to avoid influence of lead time bias in reporting of OS. The aim of the treatment for patients with PCNSL-O could be to prolong interval A (PFS) or prolong interval B (OS) or both

Instead, evaluation of secondary outcomes such as PFS should be reflective of the natural history of the disease, preferably defined as intercompartmental progression, defined as time from treatment initiation to disease progression into progression refers to involvement of the previously unaffected compartment such as ocular to CNS involvement or vice versa. Based upon the natural history of PCNSL-O, intercompartmental progression is an important event for capturing PFS, a critical outcome measure to assess overall the impact of ocular therapy. An intervention that prolongs PFS can be expected to improve OS, as death from PCNSL-O is due to CNS progression. The interest in PFS also stems in part from the fact that some treatment strategies are aimed only toward stabilization of the disease, thereby reducing the morbidity. Trials that report PFS may be conducted more quickly using fewer subjects and at lower costs than those incorporating OS [35].

Tertiary Outcome: Overall Survival (OS)

The OS is defined as the duration from diagnosis until death. In patients presenting with PCNSL-O, it would be more accurate and meaningful to report PFS (time to CNS progression) as the death in PCNSL-O is due to CNS progression. Hence, reporting of OS in these patients can be misleading unless time to CNS progression (PFS) is also reported to adjust for lead time bias (Fig. 1.1). It is important to emphasize that mere improvement of PFS does not always translate to an increase in OS, hence the great importance of analyzing OS outcomes.

Conclusions

The ultimate goal of any treatment approach in patients of PCNSL-O is to achieve long term local control, prevent progression into CNS compartments, and improve overall survival. Current literature does not conclusively support superiority or inferiority of ocular therapy compared to systemic therapy for treatment of PCNSL-O [10, 36]. In view of the increased likelihood of subsequent CNS progression, the role of adjuvant systemic chemotherapy needs to be explored in clinical trials with well-defined outcome measures.

References

1. Abrey LE, Ben-Porat L, Panageas KS, et al. Primary central nervous system lymphoma: the Memorial Sloan-Kettering Cancer Center prognostic model. J Clin Oncol. 2006;24(36):5711–5.

2. Aronow ME, Ahluwalia MS, Peereboom DM, Singh AD. Primary central nervous system and retinal lymphoma. In: Singh AD, Damato BE, editors. Clinical ophthalmic oncology retinal tumors, vol. 5. Cham: Springer-Nature; 2019.
3. Doolittle ND, Abrey LE, Shenkier TN, et al. Brain parenchyma involvement as isolated central nervous system relapse of systemic non-Hodgkin lymphoma: an International Primary CNS Lymphoma Collaborative Group report. Blood. 2008;111(3):1085–93.
4. Sorger K. Recticulum cell sarcoma of the central nervous system. Can Med Assoc J. 1963;89(10):503–7.
5. Russell DS, Marshall AH, Smith FB. Microgliomatosis; a form of reticulosis affecting the brain. Brain. 1948;71(1):1–15.
6. Cunningham ET, Miserocchi E, Smith JR, et al. Intraocular lymphoma. Ocul Immunol Inflamm. 2021;29(3):425–9.
7. Coupland SE, Damato B. Understanding intraocular lymphomas. Clin Exp Ophthalmol. 2008;36(6):564–78.
8. Takase H, Arai A, Iwasaki Y, et al. Challenges in the diagnosis and management of vitreoretinal lymphoma – clinical and basic approaches. Prog Retin Eye Res. 2022;90:101053.
9. Aziz HA, Peereboom DM, Singh AD. Primary central nervous system lymphoma. Int Ophthalmol Clin. 2015;55(1):111–21.
10. Raval V, Binkley E, Aronow ME, et al. Primary central nervous system lymphoma - ocular variant: an interdisciplinary review on management. Surv Ophthalmol. 2021;66(6):1009–20.
11. Grimm KE, O'Malley DP. Aggressive B cell lymphomas in the 2017 revised WHO classification of tumors of hematopoietic and lymphoid tissues. Ann Diagn Pathol. 2019;38:6–10.
12. Farrall AL, Smith JR. Eye involvement in primary central nervous system lymphoma. Surv Ophthalmol. 2020;65(5):548–61.
13. Chan CC, Rubenstein JL, Coupland SE, et al. Primary vitreoretinal lymphoma: a report from an International Primary Central Nervous System Lymphoma Collaborative Group Symposium. Oncologist. 2011;16(11):1589–99.
14. Hochberg FH, Miller DC. Primary central nervous system lymphoma. J Neurosurg. 1988;68(6):835–53.
15. Sagoo MS, Mehta H, Swampillai AJ, et al. Primary intraocular lymphoma. Surv Ophthalmol. 2014;59(5):503–16.
16. Hashida N, Nakai K, Saitoh N, Nishida K. Association between ocular findings and preventive therapy with onset of central nervous system involvement in patients with primary vitreoretinal lymphoma. Graefes Arch Clin Exp Ophthalmol. 2014;252(4):687–93.
17. Rali A, Xu LT, Craven C, et al. Diagnostic retinal biopsy in the management of secondary non-CNS vitreoretinal lymphoma masquerading as viral retinitis: a case report. Int J Retina Vitreous. 2021;7(1):58.
18. Reddy V, Winslow R, Cao JH, et al. Vitreoretinal lymphoma, secondary to non-CNS systemic lymphoma, masquerading as an infectious retinitis. Am J Ophthalmol Case Rep. 2019;16:100545.
19. Coupland SE, Foss HD, Assaf C, et al. T-cell and T/natural killer-cell lymphomas involving ocular and ocular adnexal tissues: a clinicopathologic, immunohistochemical, and molecular study of seven cases. Ophthalmology. 1999;106(11):2109–20.
20. Levy-Clarke GA, Greenman D, Sieving PC, et al. Ophthalmic manifestations, cytology, immunohistochemistry, and molecular analysis of intraocular metastatic T-cell lymphoma: report of a case and review of the literature. Surv Ophthalmol. 2008;53(3):285–95.
21. Bhat PV, Jakobiec FA, Papaliodis G, Sobrin L. Primary T-cell lymphoma of the retina and cerebellum: immunophenotypic and gene rearrangement confirmation. Am J Ophthalmol. 2009;148(3):350–60.
22. Chaput F, Amer R, Baglivo E, et al. Intraocular T-cell lymphoma: clinical presentation, diagnosis, treatment, and outcome. Ocul Immunol Inflamm. 2017;25(5):639–48.
23. Kamoi K, Okayama A, Izumo S, et al. Adult T-cell leukemia/lymphoma-related ocular manifestations: analysis of the first large-scale nationwide survey. Front Microbiol. 2019;9:3240.
24. Raval V, Binkley E, Aronow ME, et al. Primary central nervous system lymphoma: inter-compartmental progression. Eur J Haematol. 2022;3(2):362–70.
25. Frenkel S, Hendler K, Siegal T, et al. Intravitreal methotrexate for treating vitreoretinal lymphoma: 10 years of experience. Br J Ophthalmol. 2008;92(3):383–8.
26. Hashida N, Ohguro N, Nishida K. Efficacy and complications of intravitreal rituximab injection for treating primary vitreoretinal lymphoma. Transl Vis Sci Technol. 2012;1(3):1.
27. Abrey LE, Batchelor TT, Ferreri AJ, et al. Report of an international workshop to standardize baseline evaluation and response criteria for primary CNS lymphoma. J Clin Oncol. 2005;23(22):5034–43.
28. Schuurhuis GJ, Heuser M, Freeman S, et al. Minimal/measurable residual disease in AML: a consensus document from the European Leukemia Net MRD Working Party. Blood. 2018;131(12):1275–91.
29. Stacey AW, Pulido JS. The concept of minimal residual disease in the treatment and staging of vitreoretinal lymphoma. Retina. 2020;40(7):1213–4.

30. Riemens A, Bromberg J, Touitou V, et al. Treatment strategies in primary vitreoretinal lymphoma: a 17-center European collaborative study. JAMA Ophthalmol. 2015;133(2):191–7.
31. Ferreri AJ, Blay JY, Reni M, et al. Relevance of intraocular involvement in the management of primary central nervous system lymphomas. Ann Oncol. 2002;13(4):531–8.
32. Grimm SA, Pulido JS, Jahnke K, et al. Primary intraocular lymphoma: an International Primary Central Nervous System Lymphoma Collaborative Group Report. Ann Oncol. 2007;18(11):1851–5.
33. Grimm SA, McCannel CA, Omuro AM, et al. Primary CNS lymphoma with intraocular involvement: International PCNSL Collaborative Group Report. Neurology. 2008;71(17):1355–60.
34. Akiyama H, Takase H, Kubo F, et al. High-dose methotrexate following intravitreal methotrexate administration in preventing central nervous system involvement of primary intraocular lymphoma. Cancer Sci. 2016;107(10):1458–64.
35. Fend F, Ferreri AJ, Coupland SE. How we diagnose and treat vitreoretinal lymphoma. Br J Haematol. 2016;173(5):680–92.
36. Soussain C, Malaise D, Cassoux N. Primary vitreoretinal lymphoma: a diagnostic and management challenge. Blood. 2021;138:1519.

Epidemiological Aspects of Intraocular Lymphoma

2

M. Sanjana, Anasua Ganguly Kapoor, and Vishal R. Raval

Introduction

Lymphomas are malignant lymphoid tumors arising as clonal proliferation of either B-lymphocytes, T-lymphocytes, or natural killer cells. Lymphomas are divided into two major categories, namely Hodgkin lymphoma (HL) and non-Hodgkin lymphoma (NHL) [1]. NHL is the most common type of ocular lymphoma [2]. Depending on the site of involvement ocular lymphoma can be either ocular adnexal or intraocular lymphoma.

Ocular Adnexal Lymphoma

Anatomic Location

Ocular adnexal lymphoma (OAL) was first reported in 1952 [3]. OAL can arise from the conjunctiva, eyelids, orbit, extraocular muscles, and lacrimal apparatus [4]. The frequency of involvement has been reported as 46–74% in the orbit, 20–33% in the conjunctiva, 25% in the lacrimal gland, and 5–20% in the eyelid [5–8]. OAL arising from extraocular muscles is extremely rare with few biopsy-proven cases reported in literature with rectus muscle being most commonly affected (73%) followed by obliques (17%) and levator (11%) [9].

Pathological Subtypes

Extranodal marginal zone B-cell lymphoma (EMZL) of mucosa-associated lymphoid tissue (MALT) type constitutes about 38–100% of OAL [10]. MALT is considered the third most common form of NHL accounting for about 6–7% of extranodal non-ophthalmic NHL. An extensive review of literature of 2211 cases of orbital lymphoma by Olsen TG et al. [11] showed 97% to be of B-cell origin and 3% of T-cell origin. Out of the B-cell lymphomas 59% were extranodal marginal zone lymphoma (EMZL), followed by diffuse large B-cell lymphoma (DLBCL) (23%), follicular lymphoma (FL) (9%), and mantle cell lymphoma (MCL) (5%). Uncommon OAL variants include plasmablastic lymphoma, NK/T-cell lymphoma, small-lymphocytic lymphoma, Burkitt lymphoma (BL), lymphoplasmacytic lymphoma, plasmacytoma, and peripheral T-cell lymphoma [12–14]. Out of the T-cell lymphomas 64% were mixed T/NK-cell origin. These results are consistent with other studies where EMZL was found to be the most common type of lymphoma [6, 15–18]. Woog et al. [19] reported eight cases with natural killer/T-cell lymphomas of the

M. Sanjana · A. G. Kapoor
Hima Bindu Yalamanchili Centre for Eye Cancer, L V Prasad Eye Institute, Vijayawada, India

V. R. Raval (✉)
Anant Bajaj Retina Institute, The Operation Eyesight Universal Institute for Eye Cancer, L V Prasad Eye Institute, Hyderabad, Telangana, India

V. R. Raval et al. (eds.), *Ocular and Adnexal Lymphoma*, Essentials in Ophthalmology,
https://doi.org/10.1007/978-3-031-24595-4_2

orbit from multicenter, and they found that ocular involvement was mostly secondary to invasion from adjacent nasal or paranasal involvement with mortality of 87.5%. In a large retrospective series including SEER data from 1973 to 2015 EMZL was the most common subtype in pediatric population (45.5%) followed by DLBCL (9.1%), B lymphoblastic lymphoma (7.3%), follicular lymphoma (5.5%), Burkitt lymphoma (5.5%), and T-cell lymphoma (1.8%) [20].

Incidence

NHL is the sixth and seventh most common malignancy among females and males, respectively, in the USA with an estimated 81,560 new cases and 20,720 deaths in 2021 [21]. NHL can develop from lymphatic nodal or extranodal (outside lymph nodes, thymus, spleen, and Waldeyer's ring) sites [10]. Non-Hodgkin's lymphoma (NHL) is comprised of 4.3% of all new cancer cases and 3.4% of all cancer deaths in the USA in 2021 [22]. Primary NHL of the ocular region represents 1–2% of all NHL and 5–15% of all extranodal sites [23, 24]. Ocular adnexal lymphoma (OAL) accounts for approximately 10% of all orbital tumors [25]. Epidemiological data on ocular and ocular adnexal lymphoma are sparse in literature. In Asian countries like Japan, Korea, and also in Europe lymphoma is the most common type of malignant orbital tumor [26–29]. The overall incidence of lymphoma has been increasing annually by 3–4% [30]. From 1975 to 2001 the incidence of ocular lymphoma saw a rapid and steady rise of 6.2% and 6.5% among white males and females, respectively [10]. Similarly, the incidence of OAL has been increasing at a rate of 3.4% in the Danish population from 1980 to 2005 [31].

Age

Ocular adnexal lymphoma is a disease seen most commonly in elderly [2, 10] with a median age of 65 years [32]. In Korean population the median age of OAL was found to be 46 years at the time of diagnosis [17, 18]. However, age distribution has also been reported to vary with lymphoma subtypes. In patients older than 50 years B-cell lymphomas (73%) are more common than T-cell Lymphomas (38%) [11]. A retrospective case series studied individuals with OAL in less than 18 years of age diagnosed between 1973 and 2015 from the database of the surveillance, epidemiology and end results where the incidence of pediatric OAL was found to be 0.12 (95% CI 0.08–0.16) per 1,000,000. Males and Blacks had higher tendency for OAL [20]. Burkitt's lymphoma, B-cell lymphoblastic lymphoma, and Hodgkin's lymphoma although rare have a high incidence among young patients [10].

Gender

Incidence data from 13 surveillance, epidemiology, and end results (SEER) areas in the USA from 1992 to 2007 showed near equal gender distribution in 1604 ophthalmic and 1565 patients with OAL with higher rates of incidence in Asians and Pacific Islanders [21]. However, overall there is a slight male predominance for OAL [2]. The gender distribution depends on the specific lymphoma subtype. High grade OAL was found to have male predominance [31]. A female predominance is found among patients with EMZL (53%) and follicular lymphoma (75%). A significant male predominance is found among patients with MCL (80%) and T-cell Lymphoma (67%) [11]. A study from Denmark showed both genders being equally affected by ophthalmic NHL, with male predominance for high grade tumors [31]. International data pertaining to racial and ethnic variation of OAL is sparse.

Laterality

A majority (90%) of OALs present as a unilateral tumor [11]. A retrospective study by Kirkegaard et al. [33, 34] has reported unilateral involvement in 90% of B-cell lymphomas, while bilateral involvement was seen in mantel cell lymphoma of conjunctiva and eyelid [35]. Bilateral disease presentation is associated with poor prognosis [11, 36, 37]. A review of literature by Olsen et al. [11] reported a total of 2211 cases of OAL out of which 92% of the T-cell lymphomas had unilateral involvement, while three cases of NKTL and one case of ATCL showed bilateral involvement.

Risk Factors

Infectious Agents

Several studies have established the relationship between microorganism infection and the possibility of lymphoma arising as a result of chronic antigenic stimulation. The common organisms isolated from MALT (or marginal zone) lymphomas of various body sites are *Helicobacter pylori* (gastric), *Borrelia burgdorferi* (skin), *Chlamydia psittaci* (ocular adnexa), *Campylobacter jejuni* (small intestine), *Achromobacter xylosoxidans* (lung), and hepatitis C virus (spleen) [38, 39]. However, possibly due to geographic variations these associations have been discordant and not confirmatory [40].

H. pylori infection association with gastric-MALT lymphoma has been documented in 90% of the cases [41]. Similar association was found in OAL most commonly associated with marginal zone B-cell lymphoma with an indolent course [42–44]. Helicobacter pylori DNA was found in four of the five conjunctival MALT lymphoma cells using PCR amplification and southern blot hybridization [43]. A recent study from Taiwan showed the prevalence rate of *H. pylori* to be 53.9% [8].

Chlamydia psitacci is the next microorganism thoroughly studied in association with OAL. Ferreri et al. [45] first studied this association and reported that the DNA of chlamydia was detected by immunochemistry and PCR analysis in 87% of the 40 specimens of MALT OAL. Similar association was found in 79% of cases in Korea by Yoo et al. [46]. A study by Chanudet et al. [47] demonstrated the association of chlamydia to be significantly higher in MALT lymphoma (22%) than in non-lymphoproliferative disorder (10%) and non-marginal zone lymphomas (9%). A study by Chan CC et al. [48] reported higher prevalence of *Chlamydia pneumoniae* in non-mucosa-associated lymphoid tissues (nMALTs) as compared with MALTs in Chinese population. Thus, the prevalence varied with different geographical locations as demonstrated by Chanudet et al. [47] who demonstrated the prevalence in different countries as follows—Germany (47%) followed by the East Coast of the USA (35%) and the Netherlands (29%), but relatively low in Italy (13%), the UK (12%), and Southern China (11%).

HCV is also suspected to play a role in the etiology of B-cell NHL [49]. One study reports nine HCV-positive patients (36%) out of 25 patients with orbital EMZL [50]. A study by Ferreri AJ et al. [51] demonstrated presence of HCV in 13% patients of OAL of MALT type associated with more disseminated disease and aggressive behavior of OAL. In Taiwan the incidence of hepatitis C infection was found to be 6.2% [8].

Other studies have reported an association of human herpesvirus-6 (HHV-6) with ophthalmic MALT lymphoma in Japan and Epstein-Barr virus (EBV) has been associated with conjunctival NK/T-cell lymphomas, orbital Burkitt lymphoma, and plasmablastic lymphoma of the orbit, and human T-cell leukemia virus type 1 (HTLV-1) has also been demonstrated in patients with orbital lymphoma [2, 11].

The association of hepatitis B virus infection in EMZL was found to be more common in Chinese than Caucasian patients due to the higher incidence of genetic abnormalities like chromosome translocation and abnormal activation of innate and adaptive immunity in Asian population as compared to Western population. A study in Taiwan demonstrated HCV association in 70% of the cases [8, 52, 53].

Autoimmune Disorders and Immunodeficiency Disorders

An increased risk of NHL is reported in patients suffering from autoimmune disorders such as Sjögren's syndrome, systemic lupus erythematosus, rheumatoid arthritis, Hashimoto's thyroiditis. In these patients B-cell lymphomas, especially DLBCL and extranodal marginal zone lymphomas are the most commonly seen, whereas gastrointestinal/cutaneous autoimmune conditions are found to be associated with T-cell lymphomas [54]. In patients with human immunodeficiency virus (HIV) infection lymphoma is found to be more common than in general population and DLBCL and BL type is seen more often [55]. The mechanism of lymphoma development in HIV was postulated to be due to the higher rate of Epstein-Barr virus infection in these patients leading to activation or genomic insertion of oncogenes from the pathogen, as well as chronic antigenic stimulation [2, 11]. Thus lymphomas in immunodeficiency conditions are usually aggressive high grade B-cell in nature involving extensive extranodal sites with typically poor prognosis.

Intraocular Lymphoma

Intraocular lymphoma is a rare malignant lymphocytic neoplasm which has two main distinct forms. Primary lymphoma can be only ocular or involving the primary central nervous system and secondary or metastatic intraocular lymphoma from systemic (visceral) lymphoma [56–59]. Primary intraocular lymphoma can also be classified based on the anatomic location primarily affected—vitreoretinal lymphoma or uveal lymphoma [60]. Primary lymphoma with or without central nervous system lymphoma is an ocular subset of primary central nervous system lymphoma (PCNSL-O) predominantly affecting the subretinal space, retina, and vitreous. Patients of PCNSL-O have CNS involvement in 60–80% of cases, while 15–25% of PCNSL patients develop ocular manifestation of lymphoma and 56–90% of primary intraocular lymphoma will develop CNS manifestations of lymphoma [61–64]. Organ involvement in intraocular lymphoma can be of four types: (1) ocular-central nervous system lymphoma (most common type—(61%)), (2) intraocular lymphoma alone (17%), (3) ocular-visceral lymphoma (17%), and (4) ocular-visceral-CNS lymphoma (5%) [57]. Intraocular lymphoma has been reported as 2% of all uveitis and 33% of masquerade syndromes [65]. Primary vitreoretinal lymphoma (PVRL) represents 1.86% of ocular malignant tumors, 4–6% of all brain tumors, and less than 1% of extranodal lymphomas [66, 67]. The incidence has been found to be 0.0047 cases per 100,000 people per year which has been decreasing in immunocompromised patients with increase in HAART therapy but there is raise in incidence in immunocompetent patients [56]. PVRLs are mostly large B-cell lymphomas, very few cases of primary T-cell PVRL have been described [68, 69]. Uveal lymphomas can be further divided into those which start as a primary disease in the uveal tract or those which occur as an ocular manifestation of systemic non-Hodgkin lymphoma [70, 71].

Incidence

The incidence of PCNSL in the USA has increased more than 30 folds in three decades with an incidence rate of 0.27 per million in 1973 to 10 per million in early 1900s as documented in National Cancer Institute Surveillance, Epidemiology, and End Results (SEER) database [72, 73]. The incidence started declining to 0.43 per 100,000 person-years between 1990 and 1994 [74] and remained stable since then at 0.46 per 100,000 person-years in 2004–2007 as documented in The Central Brain Tumor Registry of the USA. This rise and subsequent stabilization of incidence is attributed to the increased incidence of human immunodeficiency virus (HIV)/AIDS and the subsequent development of highly active antiretroviral therapies (HAART). The incidence of PCNSL declined from 5.33 per 1000 person-years between 1991 and 1994 (pre-HAART) to 0.32 per 1000 person-years after 1999 (post-HAART) [75, 76]. However, this increased incidence has not been consistently observed in all geographic locations [77–79].

Risk Factors

Age

Primary intraocular lymphoma is usually seen in elderly age group. Reduced immunity and increase in number of somatic mutations can make the advancing age one of the risk factors for intraocular lymphoma [80]. The peak incidence of PCNSL is seen between 75 and 84 years, while PVRL is seen in elderly patients with a median age of 50–60 years with a range between 15 and 85 years [71, 72]. A recent case series from Singapore showed the mean age of presentation as 60.3 years [60]. While immunocompromised people at the age of 30 were also found to be affected by PCNSL [72].

Gender

PCNSL shows a male predominance with a male:female ratio of 1.38, while a female predominance is seen in PVRL with a ratio of 2:1 [71, 72]. A recent case series also reported the same female predominance of PVRL where out of nine patients five patients were females [60].

Ethnicity

Few studies state that there is no racial preference for intraocular lymphoma, while few studies show that blacks of age less than 50 years and elderly whites age more than 50 years showed higher incidence of PCNSL [72, 81]. This difference is thought to be due to more incidence of HIV/AIDS in young adults and blacks more than any other race groups in the USA [82]. In Asian population the Chinese have higher incidence of intraocular lymphoma as compared to others as reported in a case series by Hah et al. [60].

Immunodeficiency

Immunodeficiency and immunosuppression are the highest risk factors for the development of intraocular lymphoma [83]. PCNSL is commonly seen in younger age groups who suffer from skin cancer and the incidence increases with the intensive immunosuppressive treatment in these patients [72]. PCNSL is reported in 2% of patients who underwent organ transplantation and 4% in patients who have congenital immune disorders [84].

Financial Disclosure None.

Conflict of Interest None.

Funding Source This work was supported by The Operation Eyesight Universal Institute for Eye Cancer and Hyderabad Eye Research Foundation, Hyderabad, India.

References

1. Campo E, Swerdlow SH, Harris NL, Pileri S, Stein H, Jaffe ES. The 2008 WHO classification of lymphoid neoplasms and beyond: evolving concepts and practical applications. Blood. 2011;117(19):5019–32.
2. Mulay K, Honavar SG. An update on ocular adnexal lymphoma. Semin Diagn Pathol. 2016;33(3):164–72. WB Saunders.
3. Margo CE, Mulla ZD. Malignant tumors of the orbit: analysis of the Florida Cancer Registry. Ophthalmology. 1998;105(1):185–90.
4. Bellerive C, Singh AD. Cancer staging. In: Singh A, Damato B, editors. Clinical ophthalmic oncology. Cham: Springer; 2019. p. 87–91.
5. McKelvie PA, McNab A, Francis IC, Fox R, O'Day J. Ocular adnexal lymphoproliferative disease: a series of 73 cases. Clin Exp Ophthalmol. 2001;29(6):387–93.
6. Coupland SE, Krause L, Delecluse HJ, Anagnostopoulos I, Foss HD, Hummel M, Bornfeld N, Lee WR, Stein H. Lymphoproliferative lesions of the ocular adnexa: analysis of 112 cases. Ophthalmology. 1998;105(8):1430–41.
7. Knowles DM, Jakobiec FA, Mcnally L, Burke JS. Lymphoid hyperplasia and malignant lymphoma occurring in the ocular adnexa (orbit, conjunctiva, and eyelids): a prospective multiparametric analysis of 108 cases during 1977 to 1987. Hum Pathol. 1990;21(9):959–73.
8. Hsu CR, Chen YY, Yao M, Wei YH, Hsieh YT, Liao SL. Orbital and ocular adnexal lymphoma: a review of epidemiology and prognostic factors in Taiwan. Eye. 2021;35(7):1946–53.
9. Watkins LM, Carter KD, Nerad JA. Ocular adnexal lymphoma of the extraocular muscles: case series from the University of Iowa and review of the literature. Ophthalmic Plast Reconstr Surg. 2011;27(6):471–6.
10. Moslehi R, Schymura MJ, Nayak S, Coles FB. Ocular adnexal non-Hodgkin's lymphoma: a review of epidemiology and risk factors. Expert Rev Ophthalmol. 2011;6(2):181–93.
11. Olsen TG, Heegaard S. Orbital lymphoma. Surv Ophthalmol. 2019;64(1):45–66.
12. Verdijk RM. An update of ocular adnexal lymphomas. Diagn Histopathol. 2015;21(1):26–33.
13. Kim JW. Extranodal natural killer/T-cell lymphoma, nasal type, of the orbit mimicking recurrent orbital cellulitis. J Craniofac Surg. 2014;25(2):509–11.
14. Bhadauria M, Ranjan P, Mishra D. Primary orbital plasmacytoma mimicking lacrimal gland tumor. Orbit. 2014;33(4):305–7.
15. Ferry JA, Fung CY, Zukerberg L, Lucarelli MJ, Hasserjian RP, Preffer FI, Harris NL. Lymphoma of the ocular adnexa: a study of 353 cases. Am J Surg Pathol. 2007;31(2):170–84.
16. Hassan WM, Alfaar AS, Bakry MS, Ezzat S. Orbital tumors in USA: difference in survival patterns. Cancer Epidemiol. 2014;38(5):515–22.

17. Cho EY, Han JJ, Ree HJ, Ko YH, Kang YK, Ahn HS, Ahn SD, Park CJ, Huh J. Clinicopathologic analysis of ocular adnexal lymphomas: extranodal marginal zone b-cell lymphoma constitutes the vast majority of ocular lymphomas among Koreans and affects younger patients. Am J Hematol. 2003;73(2):87–96.
18. Oh DE, Kim YD. Lymphoproliferative diseases of the ocular adnexa in Korea. Arch Ophthalmol. 2007;125(12):1668–73.
19. Woog JJ, Kim YD, Yeatts RP, Kim S, Esmaeli B, Kikkawa D, Lee HH, Korn BS, Punja K, Habermann TM, Colgan JP. Natural killer/T-cell lymphoma with ocular and adnexal involvement. Ophthalmology. 2006;113(1):140–7.
20. Moustafa GA, Topham AK, Aronow ME, Vavvas DG. Paediatric ocular adnexal lymphoma: a population-based analysis. BMJ Open Ophthalmol. 2020;5(1):e000483.
21. American Cancer Society. Cancer facts and figures 2021. Atlanta, GA: American Cancer Society; 2021.
22. Miller KD, Nogueira L, Mariotto AB, Rowland JH, Yabroff KR, Alfano CM, Jemal A, Kramer JL, Siegel RL. Cancer treatment and survivorship statistics, 2019. CA Cancer J Clin. 2019;69(5):363–85.
23. Fitzpatrick PJ, Macko S. Lymphoreticular tumors of the orbit. Int J Radiat Oncol Biol Phys. 1984;10(3):333–40.
24. Freeman C, Berg JW, Cutler SJ. Occurrence and prognosis of extranodal lymphomas. Cancer. 1972;29(1):252–60.
25. Rubinstein TJ, Aziz HA, Bellerive C, Sires BS, Hing AW, Habermehl G, Hsi E, Singh AD. Ocular/adnexal lymphoma: dissimilar to systemic lymphoma. Surv Ophthalmol. 2018;63(3):381–8.
26. Ohtsuka K, Hashimoto M, Suzuki Y. High incidence of orbital malignant lymphoma in Japanese patients. Am J Ophthalmol. 2004;138(5):881–2.
27. Shikishima K, Kawai K, Kitahara K. Pathological evaluation of orbital tumours in Japan: analysis of a large case series and 1379 cases reported in the Japanese literature. Clin Exp Ophthalmol. 2006;34(3):239–44.
28. Ko YH, Kim CW, Park CS, Jang HK, Lee SS, Kim SH, et al. REAL classification of malignant lymphomas in the Republic of Korea: incidence of recently recognized entities and changes in clinicopathologic features. Hematolymphoreticular Study Group of the Korean Society of Pathologists. Revised European-American lymphoma. Cancer. 1998;83(4):806–12.
29. Seregard S, Sahlin S. Panorama of orbital space-occupying lesions. The 24-year experience of a referral centre. Acta Ophthalmol Scand. 1999;77(1):91–8.
30. Clarke CA, Glaser SL. Changing incidence of non-Hodgkin lymphomas in the United States. Cancer. 2002;94(7):2015–23.
31. Sjo LD, Ralfkiaer E, Prause JU, Petersen JH, Madsen J, Pedersen NT, Heegaard S. Increasing incidence of ophthalmic lymphoma in Denmark from 1980 to 2005. Invest Ophthalmol Vis Sci. 2008;49(8):3283–8.
32. Sjö LD. Ophthalmic lymphoma: epidemiology and pathogenesis. Acta Ophthalmol. 2009;87(1):1–20.
33. Kirkegaard MM, Coupland SE, Prause JU, Heegaard S. Malignant lymphoma of the conjunctiva. Surv Ophthalmol. 2015;60(5):444–58.
34. Kirkegaard MM, Rasmussen PK, Coupland SE, et al. Conjunctival lymphoma--an international multicenter retrospective study. JAMA Ophthalmol. 2016;134(4):406–14.
35. Svendsen FH, Heegaard S. Lymphoma of the eyelid. Surv Ophthalmol. 2017;62(3):312–31.
36. Jenkins C, Rose GE, Bunce C, Cree I, Norton A, Plowman PN, et al. Clinical features associated with survival of patients with lymphoma of the ocular adnexa. Eye. 2003;17:809–20.
37. Desai A, Joag MG, Lekakis L, Chapman JR, Vega F, Tibshirani R, et al. Long-term course of patients with primary ocular adnexal MALT lymphoma: a large single-institution cohort study. Blood. 2017;129:324–32.
38. Inagaki H. Mucosa-associated lymphoid tissue lymphoma: molecular pathogenesis and clinicopathological significance. Pathol Int. 2007;57(8):474–84.
39. Verdijk RM. Lymphoproliferative tumors of the ocular adnexa. Asia Pac J Ophthalmol. 2017;6(2):132–42.
40. Zucca E, Bertoni F. The spectrum of MALT lymphoma at different sites: biological and therapeutic relevance. Blood. 2016;127(17):2082–92.
41. Wotherspoon AC, Ortiz-Hidalgo C, Falzon MR, Isaacson PG. Helicobacter pylori-associated gastritis and primary B-cell gastric lymphoma. Lancet. 1991;338(8776):1175–6.
42. Verma V, Shen D, Sieving PC, Chan CC. The role of infectious agents in the etiology of ocular adnexal neoplasia. Surv Ophthalmol. 2008;53(4):312–31.
43. Chan CC, Smith JA, Shen D, Ursea R, LeHoang P, Grossniklaus HE. Helicobacter pylori (H. pylori) molecular signature in conjunctival mucosa-associated lymphoid tissue (MALT) lymphoma. Histol Histopathol. 2004;19(4):1219.
44. Ferreri AJ, Ponzoni M, Viale E, Guidoboni M, Conciliis CD, Resti AG, Politi L, Lettini AA, Sacchetti F, Dognini G, Dolcetti R. Association between Helicobacter pylori infection and MALT-type lymphoma of the ocular adnexa: clinical and therapeutic implications. Hematol Oncol. 2006;24(1):33–7.
45. Ferreri AJ, Guidoboni M, Ponzoni M, De Conciliis C, Dell'Oro S, Fleischhauer K, Caggiari L, Lettini AA, Dal Cin E, Ieri R, Freschi M. Evidence for an association between Chlamydia psittaci and ocular adnexal lymphomas. J Natl Cancer Inst. 2004;96(8):586–94.
46. Yoo C, Ryu MH, Huh J, Park JH, Kang HJ, Ahn HS, Lee Y, Kim MJ, Lee H, Kim TW, Chang HM. Chlamydia psittaci infection and clinicopathologic analysis of ocular adnexal lymphomas in Korea. Am J Hematol. 2007;82(9):821–3.
47. Chanudet E, Zhou Y, Bacon CM, Wotherspoon AC, Müller-Hermelink HK, Adam P, Dong HY, De Jong D, Li Y, Wei R, Gong X. Chlamydia psittaci is vari-

ably associated with ocular adnexal MALT lymphoma in different geographical regions. J Pathol. 2006;209(3):344–51.
48. Chan CC, Shen D, Mochizuki M, Gonzales JA, Yuen HK, Guex-Crosier Y, LeHoang P. Detection of Helicobacter pylori and Chlamydia pneumoniae genes in primary orbital lymphoma. Trans Am Ophthalmol Soc. 2006;104:62.
49. Ascoli V, Coco FL, Artini M, Levrero M, Martelli M, Negro F. Extranodal lymphomas associated with hepatitis C virus infection. Am J Clin Pathol. 1998;109(5):600–9.
50. Arcaini L, Burcheri S, Rossi A, Paulli M, Bruno R, Passamonti F, Brusamolino E, Molteni A, Pulsoni A, Cox MC, Orsucci L. Prevalence of HCV infection in nongastric marginal zone B-cell lymphoma of MALT. Ann Oncol. 2007;18(2):346–50.
51. Ferreri AJ, Viale E, Guidoboni M, Resti AG, De Conciliis C, Politi L, Lettini AA, Sacchetti F, Dolcetti R, Doglioni C, Ponzoni M. Clinical implications of hepatitis C virus infection in MALT-type lymphoma of the ocular adnexa. Ann Oncol. 2006;17(5):769–72.
52. Chuang SS, Lee C, Hamoudi RA, Liu H, Lee PS, Ye H, Diss TC, Dogan A, Isaacson PG, Du MQ. High frequency of t (11; 18) in gastric mucosa-associated lymphoid tissue lymphomas in Taiwan, including one patient with high-grade transformation. Br J Haematol. 2003;120(1):97–100.
53. Tanimoto K, Kaneko A, Suzuki S, Sekiguchi N, Watanabe T, Kobayashi Y, Kagami Y, Maeshima AM, Matsuno Y, Tobinai K. Primary ocular adnexal MALT lymphoma: a long-term follow-up study of 114 patients. Jpn J Clin Oncol. 2007;37(5):337–44.
54. Mendes LS, Wotherspoon A. Marginal zone lymphoma: associated autoimmunity and auto-immune disorders. Best Pract Res Clin Haematol. 2017;30(1–2):65–76.
55. Riedel DJ, Rositch AF, Redfield RR, Blattner WA. HIV-associated lymphoma sub-type distribution, immunophenotypes and survival in an urban clinic population. Leuk Lymphoma. 2016;57(2):306–12.
56. Sagoo MS, Mehta H, Swampillai AJ, Cohen VM, Amin SZ, Plowman PN, Lightman S. Primary intraocular lymphoma. Surv Ophthalmol. 2014;59(5):503–16.
57. Raval V, Binkley E, Aronow ME, Valenzuela J, Peereboom DM, Singh AD. Primary central nervous system lymphoma - ocular variant: an interdisciplinary review on management. Surv Ophthalmol. 2021;66(6):1009–20.
58. Cooper EL, Riker JL. Malignant lymphoma of the uveal tract. Am J Ophthalmol. 1951;34(8):1153–8.
59. Givner I. Malignant lymphoma with ocular involvement: a clinico-pathologic report. Am J Ophthalmol. 1955;39(1):29–32.
60. Hah YY, Ho SL, Beng SC, Agrawal R. Epidemiology and clinical features of intraocular lymphoma in Singapore. Nepal J Ophthalmol. 2019;11(22):158–66.
61. Akpek EK, Ahmed I, Hochberg FH, Soheilian M, Dryja TP, Jakobiec FA, Foster CS. Intraocular-central nervous system lymphoma: clinical features, diagnosis, and outcomes. Ophthalmology. 1999;106(9):1805–10.
62. Chan CC. Molecular pathology of primary intraocular lymphoma. Trans Am Ophthalmol Soc. 2003;101:275.
63. Peterson K, Gordon KB, Heinemann MH, DeAngelis LM. The clinical spectrum of ocular lymphoma. Cancer. 1993;72(3):843–9.
64. DeAngelis LM, Hormigo A. Treatment of primary central nervous system lymphoma. Semin Oncol. 2004;31(5):684–92. WB Saunders.
65. Rothova A, Ooijman F, Kerkhoff F, et al. Uveitis masquerade syndromes. Ophthalmology. 2001;108(2):386–99.
66. Coupland SE, Damato B. Understanding intraocular lymphomas. Clin Exp Ophthalmol. 2008;36(6):564–78.
67. Chan CC, Rubenstein JL, Coupland SE, Davis JL, Harbour JW, Johnston PB, Cassoux N, Touitou V, Smith JR, Batchelor TT, Pulido JS. Primary vitreoretinal lymphoma: a report from an international primary central nervous system lymphoma collaborative group symposium. Oncologist. 2011;16(11):1589.
68. Schabet M. Epidemiology of primary CNS lymphoma. J Neuro-Oncol. 1999;43(3):199–201.
69. Olson JE, Janney CA, Rao RD, Cerhan JR, Kurtin PJ, Schiff D, Kaplan RS, O'Neill BP. The continuing increase in the incidence of primary central nervous system non-Hodgkin lymphoma: a surveillance, epidemiology, and end results analysis. Cancer. 2002;95(7):1504–10.
70. Surawicz TS, McCarthy BJ, Kupelian V, Jukich PJ, Bruner JM, Davis FG. Descriptive epidemiology of primary brain and CNS tumors: results from the Central Brain Tumor Registry of the United States, 1990-1994. Neuro-Oncology. 1999;1(1):14–25.
71. Coupland SE, Heimann H, Bechrakis NE. Primary intraocular lymphoma: a review of the clinical, histopathological and molecular biological features. Graefes Arch Clin Exp Ophthalmol. 2004;242:901–13.
72. Villano JL, Koshy M, Shaikh H, Dolecek TA, McCarthy BJ. Age, gender, and racial differences in incidence and survival in primary CNS lymphoma. Br J Cancer. 2011;105(9):1414–8.
73. Yoon JS, Lee CS, Lee S. Ocular and adnexal lymphoma: epidemiological aspects. In: Singh A, editor. Ocular and adnexal lymphoma. Berlin: Springer; 2014. p. 47–56.
74. Hao D, DiFrancesco LM, Brasher PM, et al. Is primary CNS lymphoma really becoming more common? A population-based study of incidence, clinicopathological features and outcomes in Alberta from 1975 to 1996. Ann Oncol. 1999;10(1):65–70.
75. Yau YH, O'Sullivan MG, Signorini D, et al. Primary lymphoma of central nervous system in immunocompetent patients in south-east Scotland. Lancet. 1996;348(9031):890.

76. Krogh-Jensen M, D'Amore F, Jensen MK, et al. Clinicopathological features, survival and prognostic factors of primary central nervous system lymphomas: trends in incidence of primary central nervous system lymphomas and primary malignant brain tumors in a well-defined geographical area. Population-based data from the Danish Lymphoma Registry, LYFO, and the Danish Cancer Registry. Leuk Lymphoma. 1995;19(3–4):223–33.
77. Reddy EK, Bhatia P, Evans RG. Primary orbital lymphomas. Int J Radiat Oncol Biol Phys. 1988;15(5):1239–41.
78. Venkatesh R, Bavaharan B, Mahendradas P, Yadav NK. Primary vitreoretinal lymphoma: prevalence, impact, and management challenges. Clin Ophthalmol. 2019;13:353.
79. Kluin PM. Primary diffuse large B-cell lymphoma of the CNS. In: Swerdlow SH, Campo E, Harris NL, editors. World Health Organization: pathology and genetics of tumors of haematopoietic and lymphoid tissues. Lyon: IARC Press; 2008. p. 240–1.
80. Coupland SE, Anastassiou G, Bornfeld N, Hummel M, Stein H. Primary intraocular lymphoma of T-cell type: report of a case and review of the literature. Graefes Arch Clin Exp Ophthalmol. 2005;243(3):189–97.
81. Fine HA, Mayer RJ. Primary central nervous system lymphoma. Ann Intern Med. 1993;119(11):1093–104.
82. Morris M, Handcock MS, Miller WC, Ford CA, Schmitz JL, Hobbs MM, Cohen MS, Harris KM, Udry JR. Prevalence of HIV infection among young adults in the United States: results from the Add Health Study. Am J Public Health. 2006;96(6):1091–7.
83. Mochizuki M, Singh AD. Epidemiology and clinical features of intraocular lymphoma. Ocul Immunol Inflamm. 2009;17(2):69–72.
84. Patchell RA. Primary central nervous system lymphoma in the transplant patient. Neurol Clin. 1988;6(2):297–303.

Ocular and Adnexal Lymphoma: Pathogenesis and Pathology

3

Sarah L. Ondrejka

Introduction

Ocular and adnexal lymphoma (OAL) refers to lymphoma involving either the orbit or the ocular adnexa. The ocular adnexa refers to tissues and structures surrounding the eye, such as conjunctiva, the lacrimal gland, the eyelids, and the surrounding orbital soft tissue. Approximately 8% of all extranodal lymphomas arise in the ocular adnexa [1]. Ocular adnexal lymphomas predominantly affect older individuals, with a median age in the 60s, and with a slight female predominance. Intraocular lymphomas are rare, representing less than 1% of all intraocular tumors and have a close association with primary central nervous system (CNS) lymphoma [2]. In this review, the histological and immunophenotypical features of the intraocular and ocular adnexal lymphomas will be discussed, and relevant molecular genetic features and pathogenesis will be briefly summarized.

Intraocular Lymphoma

Intraocular lymphoma is a subset of primary CNS lymphoma that may occur synchronously with lymphoma in the brain or is an isolated abnormality. Of all patients with primary CNS lymphoma, approximately 10–25% have ocular involvement. Patients with intraocular diffuse large B-cell lymphoma have a high risk of developing contralateral tumors (approximately 80%) or associated parenchymal central nervous system lesions [3]. Vitreoretinal lymphoma is another term used to refer to these high-grade intraocular malignancies. PCNSL-O is the preferred term to emphasize that it is an ocular variant or subset of primary CNS lymphoma (PCNSL).

To establish a diagnosis of lymphoma, patients may undergo vitrectomy, choroidal/retinal biopsy, or vitreous aspiration. In some cases, tailoring the biopsy approach in order to obtain fresh tissue for flow cytometry can be helpful to establish a clonal B-cell population [4]. The immunoglobulin genes are clonally rearranged and heavily somatically mutated, al1though demonstrating an immunoglobulin heavy chain or kappa region gene rearrangement is not a necessity for making the diagnosis [5, 6]. Determining the IL-10 and IL-6 levels in the vitreous may be helpful in evaluating the possibility of lymphoma since an elevated IL-10 level in the vitreous is strongly associated with ocular lymphoma. As a growth and differentiation factor for B cells, IL-10 promotes proliferation of neoplastic B cells and serves as an immunosuppressive cytokine that protects the lymphoma cells from the immune system. IL-6 may be released by the

S. L. Ondrejka (✉)
Robert J. Tomsich Pathology & Laboratory Medicine Institute, Cleveland Clinic, Cleveland, OH, USA
e-mail: ondrejs@ccf.org

V. R. Raval et al. (eds.), *Ocular and Adnexal Lymphoma*, Essentials in Ophthalmology,
https://doi.org/10.1007/978-3-031-24595-4_3

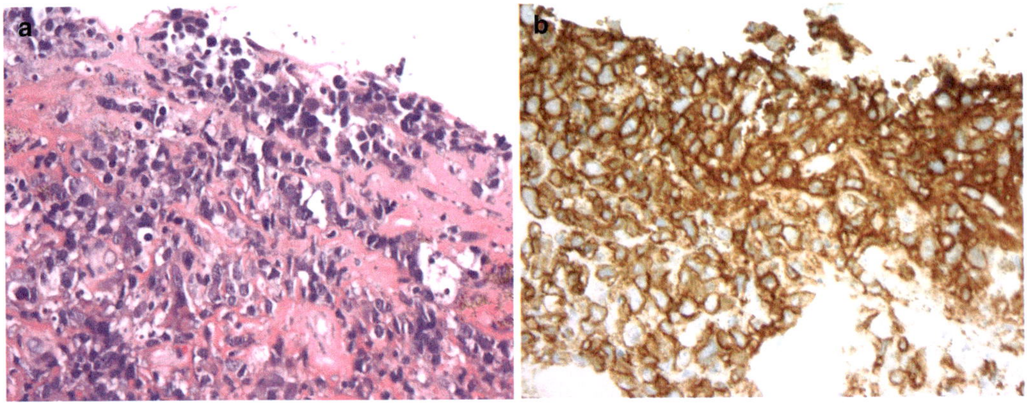

Fig. 3.1 Diffuse large B-cell lymphoma involving the choroid and retina. (**a**) There is a diffuse infiltrate of large neoplastic lymphocytes with irregular nuclear contours and hyperchromatic chromatin with occasional small nucleoli (400×, H&E). (**b**) The cells are diffusely positive for CD20 (400×, CD20)

reactive inflammatory population in cases of ocular lymphoma. An elevated IL-10 to IL-6 ratio suggests lymphoma rather than inflammation, but may not be elevated in early stages of lymphoma [6, 7].

Microscopically, the retina or optic nerve shows a diffuse perivascular infiltrate of large transformed lymphoid cells, with round or ovoid nuclei, nuclear membrane irregularities, high nuclear to cytoplasmic ratios, and prominent nucleoli (Fig. 3.1). Early in the course of disease, neoplastic cells can be found between Bruch's membrane and the retinal pigment epithelium [8]. Cytologic evaluation of the vitreous shows large pleomorphic lymphoid cells with nucleoli. Mitotic figures are easily identified. Necrosis and apoptosis with tingible body macrophages are present in highly proliferative lesions (Fig. 3.2).

The usual immunophenotype is characterized by positivity for B-cell antigens (CD20, CD79a, PAX 5), as well as positivity for MUM1, BCL2, BCL6, and usually monotypic IgM (Fig. 3.1). CD10 expression is much less common and could indicate secondary involvement by systemic diffuse large B-cell lymphoma. The tumors are Epstein-Barr virus negative. In immunocompetent patients, the histogenesis and immunophenotypic features correspond to the late germinal center or early post-germinal center stage of differentiation, quite similar to primary CNS lymphoma in the brain. Combining the non-germinal

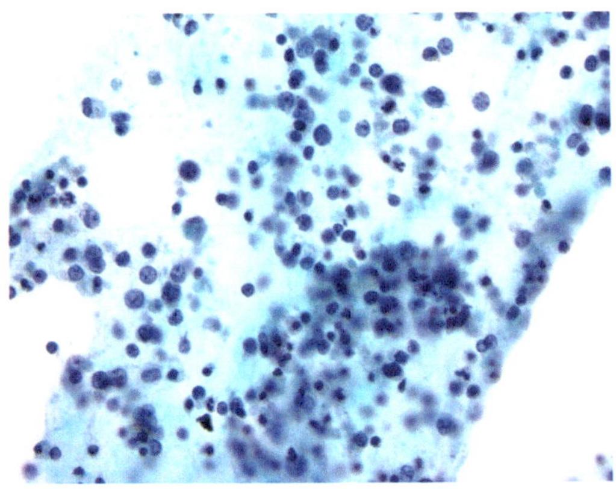

Fig. 3.2 Eye fine needle aspiration of vitreous showing an abnormal population of large lymphoid cells consistent with diffuse large B-cell lymphoma (400×, Thin-prep)

center immunophenotype (CD10−/BCL6+/−/MUM1+) by the Hans algorithm with the high somatic mutation load in the immunoglobulin variable region, this points to a histogenetic cell of origin corresponding to the activated B-cell-like subtype of diffuse large B-cell lymphoma by gene expression profiling [9–12].

Primary Uveal Lymphoma

Primary lymphoid proliferations of the uvea are rare and usually occur as primary choroidal lymphoma. Primary ciliary body lymphoma and primary iridal lymphoma are less common. Primary choroidal lymphoma was thought to be erroneously a form of reactive lymphoid hyperplasia in earlier literature, but subsequent study has shown that these have clinical and pathologic features of extranodal marginal zone lymphoma of mucosa-associated lymphoid tissue [13, 14]. Grossly, these lymphomas demonstrate diffuse thickening of the choroid that may result in retinal detachment. In some cases the overlying conjunctiva is involved, but overall changes occur slowly reflective of the indolent disease process [15].

Cytologic specimens will show a monotonous proliferation of small lymphocytes. Histologic biopsies show features of extranodal marginal zone lymphoma including a heterogeneous proliferation of centrocyte-like and monocytoid B cells, and occasional immunoblasts and plasmacytoid cells. Mitoses are infrequent. Lymphoepithelial lesions, or what has been described as the "uveal equivalent" can be seen as small lymphoma cells invading Bruch's membrane and the retinal epithelium [16]. Lymphoepithelial lesions are characteristic of marginal zone lymphomas of MALT type and are defined as aggregates of marginal zone B cells with distortion or distraction of the epithelium or glandular tissue [17]. Immunophenotypic studies demonstrate a light-chain restricted B-cell phenotype positive for CD20, CD79a, and PAX5 and usually negative for CD5, CD10, and cyclinD1 [16, 17].

Primary iridal lymphoma is extremely rare and demonstrates high-grade cytology. It is a cause of steroid-resistant uveitis in patients who usually have a history of an aggressive systemic B-cell lymphoma. Iris biopsies demonstrate sheets of large atypical transformed lymphocytes with pleomorphic cytology, frequent mitoses, and a high Ki-67 proliferative fraction [18]. In most cases, iridal involvement represents secondary iris infiltration by primary intraocular lymphoma, and the extent of iridal involvement is not documented until enucleation or post-mortem examination [19].

Secondary intraocular involvement by lymphoma involves spread to the eye by systemic lymphoma involving extranodal or lymph node primary sites. This usually arises by hematologic spread to the uvea and most commonly occurs as extension by primary CNS lymphoma, though many other systemic lymphomas have been reported including diffuse large B-cell lymphoma, some types of T-cell lymphoma, and lymphoblastic lymphomas [9].

Ocular Adnexal Lymphoma

Ocular adnexal lymphomas represent approximately 8% of extranodal lymphomas and are composed of several different subtypes. It is a disease of older adults with a slight female predominance. The prognosis largely depends upon the histologic diagnosis, with favorable outcomes in low-grade B-cell lesions such as extranodal marginal zone lymphoma (ENMZL) and follicular lymphoma [1]. Other subtypes of lymphoma known to occur in the ocular adnexa include mantle cell lymphoma (MCL), small lymphocytic lymphoma (SLL), lymphoplasmacytic lymphoma (LPL), splenic marginal zone lymphoma (SMZL), diffuse large B-cell lymphoma, not otherwise specified, lymphoblastic lymphoma, peripheral T-cell lymphoma, and extranodal NK/T-cell lymphoma, nasal type. Classic Hodgkin lymphoma is exceedingly rare and occurs as a secondary manifestation. Marginal zone lymphoma usually involves the ocular adnexa as a primary site, with fewer cases of follicular lymphoma and diffuse large B-cell lymphoma arising as ocular adnexal primaries, and the other listed subtypes may involve the ocular adnexa secondarily [20]. Of patients with non-Hodgkin lymphoma, approximately 5% will develop secondary ocular adnexal involvement during the course of their disease [21]. This section describes the histologic, immunophenotypic, and genetic findings of some of the more common types of non-Hodgkin lymphoma involving the ocular adnexa.

Extranodal Marginal Zone Lymphoma (ENMZL) of Mucosa-Associated Lymphoid Tissue (MALT)

ENMZL was first described in the stomach but can arise in a variety of extranodal sites. These are indolent lymphomas that usually arise from mucosa-associated lymphoid tissue that accumulates as a result of a chronic inflammatory disorder, chronic antigenic stimulation, and/or autoimmunity. ENMZL is often referred to as "MALT" lymphomas when involving overlying epithelium such as conjunctiva or lacrimal gland acinar structures, but this designation is not appropriate when referring to marginal zone lymphomas involving areas deep within the orbit [22].

Histologic findings in ENMZL of the ocular adnexa include mass-forming infiltrates of small to medium-sized irregular lymphoplasmacytic infiltrates, residual foci of follicular center cells, and lymphoepithelial lesions in areas where there is overlying epithelium (Fig. 3.3a, b). There are rare to few mitoses. Dutcher bodies and polykaryocytes are sometimes identified [20]. One study of histologic characteristics showed that some features that are typical of ENMZL-MALT at other sites including monocytoid cytology, plasmacytoid differentiation, and lymphoepithelial lesions are less common in ENMZL affecting the ocular adnexa [23].

The immunophenotype of ENMZL is reflective of the histogenetic origin as marginal zone B cells (Fig. 3.3c). The lymphomas are positive for CD19, CD20, CD79a and often aberrantly express CD43 (a T-cell marker) and BCL2 (Fig. 3.3). There is restricted surface immunoglobulin expression that can be demonstrated by flow cytometry. CD21 positive follicular dendritic cell meshworks are sometimes expanded or disrupted by the infiltrate. Plasmacytic differentiation can be demonstrated by Dutcher bodies and immunoglobulin deposits and immunohistochemistry for kappa and lambda demonstrating

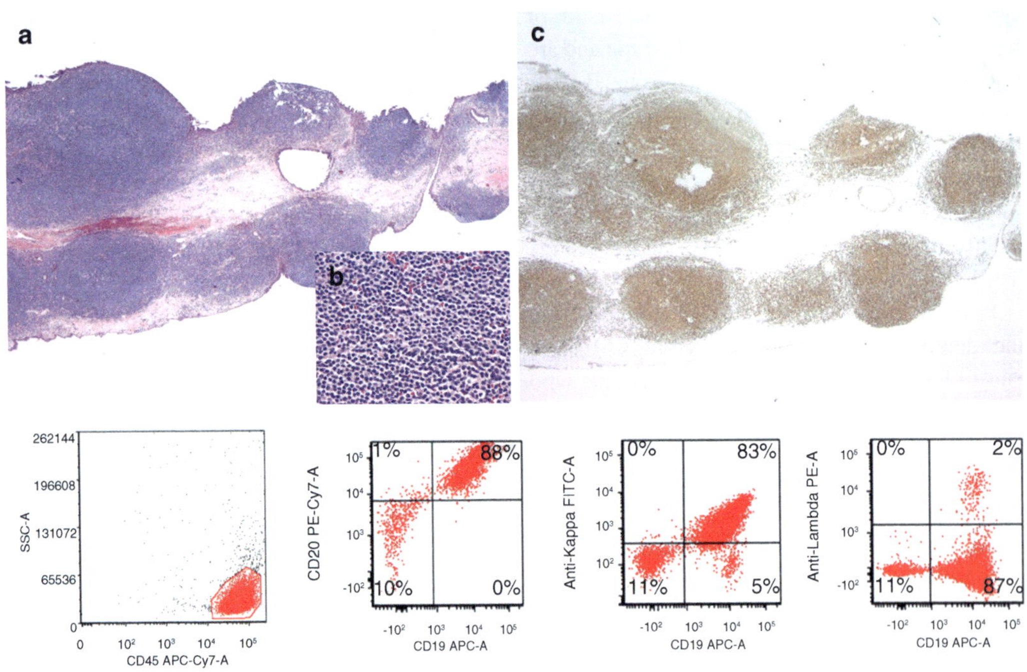

Fig. 3.3 Extranodal marginal zone lymphoma of mucosa-associated lymphoid tissue. (**a**) There are diffuse and nodular aggregates of lymphoma associated with the conjunctiva epithelium (10×, H&E). (**b**) The cells are monotonous with moderate cytoplasm and there is a circumscribed focus of larger cells toward the right edge of the photograph consistent with a residual follicle (400×, H&E). (**c**) The infiltrate is composed of excess B cells (400×, CD20). The lower row of images are flow cytometry plots. The analysis shows a uniform lymphoid population positive for CD19, CD20, and monotypic kappa surface immunoglobulin

monotypic cytoplasmic immunoglobulin [24] (Fig. 3.3). CD5 is rarely expressed, and cyclinD1 is negative. IRTA1 is a newer marker that was developed to assist in the differential diagnosis of marginal zone lymphomas. It is expressed by monocytoid B cells, marginal zone cells, and intraepithelial B cells in normal tissues and was demonstrated to be a helpful, specific marker in identification of ENMZL when present, though has limited sensitivity [25].

Flow cytometry or molecular methods are essential in the differential diagnosis of ENMZL from reactive lymphoid hyperplasia. Earlier studies of lymphoproliferative lesions identified histologic criteria to separate reactive lymphoid hyperplasia at one end of the histologic spectrum from other B-cell lymphoma types, but demonstrating a clonal population by light chain restriction or PCR is optimal for diagnosis [24]. Immunoglobulin heavy-chain and light-chain genes are clonally rearranged and can be demonstrated with testing using BIOMED-2/EuroClonality consensus primer sets, which detect a clonal population in approximately 85% of cases [26].

In order for flow cytometry to be performed, biopsies must be of sufficient size to allow for morphologic review and to allow for a single cell suspension to be derived from processing of fresh tissue. A portion of the specimen must be sent fresh or in supportive media to the performing laboratory within time requirements for stability. If flow cytometry is not performed, it can be difficult to detect light chains in neoplastic lymphocytes using tissue sections alone. However, recent data employing newer techniques for ultrasensitive detection of kappa and lambda using a RNA-based in situ hybridization method has shown results comparable or superior to flow cytometry. In a study of tissue biopsies fixed in formalin, RNA in situ hybridization identified light-chain restricted B cells in 89% of B-cell lymphomas compared to 67% of B-cell lymphomas by flow cytometry [27].

Several genetic abnormalities have been described in ENMZL/MALT lymphoma, including trisomy of chromosome 3 and chromosome 18 in slightly over half of cases. Gains of chromosome 3 are found more frequently in orbital cases compared with lymphomas involving the lacrimal gland [23, 28]. Recurrent translocations include t(11;18)(q21;q21)/*BIRC3::MALT1*, t(1;14)(p22;q32)/*BCL10::IGH*, t(14;18)(q32;q21)/*IGH::MALT1*, and t(3;14)(p13;q32)/*FOXP1::IGH* [29–31]. The oncogenic products of the first three translocations cause NF-κB activation. In MALT lymphomas lacking the above translocations, array comparative hybridization identified that the A20 gene, an inhibitor of NF-κB activity, was inactivated by somatic deletion or mutation in ocular adnexal ENMZL [32]. Details of recurrent chromosomal abnormalities in ENMZL are found in Table 3.1.

Table 3.1 Cytogenetic and molecular genetic abnormalities in ocular adnexal extranodal marginal zone lymphoma

Structural abnormality	Genes involved	Frequency (%)
+3		38%
+18		13%
t(11;18)(q21;q21)	*BIRC3, MALT1*	0–10%
t(14;18)(p14;q32)	*IGH, MALT1*	7–25%
t(3;14)(p22;q32)	*IGH, FOXP1*	0–20%

Pathogenesis and Etiology

ENMZLs arise in lymphoid tissue in extranodal sites as a result of chronic inflammation due to antigen stimulation and sometimes autoimmune disorders. For example, there is strong evidence that gastric MALT lymphoma and infection with *Helicobacter pylori* are closely linked. The significance of *C. psittaci* infection to development of ENMZL of the ocular adnexa is still unclear. In 2004, a high association between this organism and conjunctival MALT lymphoma was demonstrated by PCR studies. Furthermore, eradication of infection with doxycycline was effective in treating the lymphoma and producing a complete response [33]. This group went on to culture *C. psittaci* in blood and conjunctiva from patients with OAL and demonstrated its absence in normal healthy controls [33]. However, subsequent studies from other groups worldwide have demonstrated significant variability in association with *C. psittaci* between regions of the world and between studies and variable efficacy of antibiotics as treatment. In general, higher prevalence rates in Italy and South Korea have been described, with a lower incidence in the USA. Lack of *C. psittaci* in some series indicates that geographic heterogeneity may be a contributing factor to differences in pathogenesis of ENMZL [23, 34].

Other Subtypes of Ocular Adnexal Lymphoma

Diffuse large B-cell lymphoma and related large B-cell lymphomas are aggressive tumors composed of transformed cells, either derived from centroblasts (germinal center like-cells) or activated B-cell-like cells committed to terminal B-cell differentiation stages [11]. Some lymphomas in this category have high-grade cytology with intermediate-sized or blastoid nuclei. These may secondarily involve the ocular adnexa and form destructive masses, but it is sometimes difficult to determine if these lymphomas arise from the orbit primarily [20]. Diffuse large B-cell lymphoma is a heterogeneous disease with many biologic factors and oncogenic mechanisms that impact response to therapy and survival, and pathologic evaluation involves, at a minimum, histologic review, cell of origin classification by immunohistochemistry, and FISH studies for additional classification and prognostication [35].

Follicular lymphoma is the second most common indolent B-cell lymphoma occurring in the ocular adnexa [20]. It is a neoplasm of malignant centrocytes and centroblasts, which are derived from the germinal center. The growth pattern can be follicular or partially follicular, but purely diffuse low-grade patterns are also recognized. Grading according to the proportion of centroblasts is used to further subclassify into categories of grade 1-2, 3A, and 3B recognized by the WHO classification. Follicular lymphoma has a distinctive immunophenotype involving expression of germinal center markers including CD10, BCL6, and MEF2B and demonstrates abnormal expression of BCL2 in most cases. The t(14;18)(q32;q21) is an early event in most cases, though translocation negative follicular lymphomas are also described. Additional genetic and epigenetic abnormalities are responsible for the pathogenesis [36].

Ocular adnexal mantle cell lymphoma more often represents secondary involvement of this region in patients with a history of mantle cell lymphoma in other extranodal sites such as the Waldeyer ring, gastrointestinal tract, and soft tissue [20]. The lymphoma is usually aggressive and presents at a high clinical stage, with frequent bilateral involvement and poor prognosis. The cells are small- to medium-sized with irregular or cleaved nuclei, and cytologically can mimic

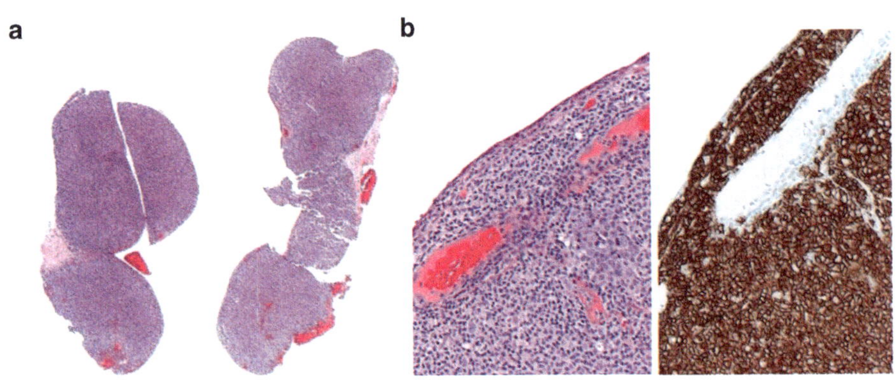

Fig. 3.4 Mantle cell lymphoma involving conjunctiva. (**a**) There are multiple nodular, expansive aggregates of lymphocytes under the epithelium (20×, H&E), composed of intermediate-sized monotonous lymphocytes with irregular nuclei (400×, inset). (**b**) The lymphocytes are positive for cyclinD1 by immunohistochemistry (20×, cyclinD1)

low-grade indolent B-cell lymphomas including MZL and follicular lymphoma (Fig. 3.4a). The lymphoma cells are positive for B-cell antigens and CD5, cyclinD1, and SOX11, with monoclonal surface immunoglobulin [37] (Fig. 3.4b).

Conclusions

Ocular and adnexal lymphomas are usually B-cell lymphomas that vary in histologic characteristics and behavior. The incidence of OAL has risen over the past several decades, increasing up to 6.5% per year according to SEER data [38]. Our understanding of lymphoma histology and biology and the molecular genetic underpinnings of the lymphoma subtypes has also grown relatively quickly in parallel, and additional studies to identify risk factors and additional pathogenetic mechanisms will be helpful for future prevention and therapy.

References

1. Freeman C, Berg JW, Cutler SJ. Occurrence and prognosis of extranodal lymphomas. Cancer. 1972;29(1):252–60.
2. Bardenstein DS. Intraocular lymphoma. Cancer Control. 1998;5(4):317–25.
3. Korfel A, Schlegel U. Diagnosis and treatment of primary CNS lymphoma. Nat Rev Neurol. 2013;9(6):317–27.
4. Wilson DJ, Braziel R, Rosenbaum JT. Intraocular lymphoma. Immunopathologic analysis of vitreous biopsy specimens. Arch Ophthalmol. 1992;110(10):1455–8.
5. Coupland SE, Hummel M, Müller H-H, Stein H. Molecular analysis of immunoglobulin genes in primary intraocular lymphoma. Invest Ophthalmol Vis Sci. 2005;46(10):3507–14.
6. Chan C-C. Molecular pathology of primary intraocular lymphoma. Trans Am Ophthalmol Soc. 2003;101:275–92.
7. Whitcup SM, Stark-Vancs V, Wittes RE, Solomon D, Podgor MJ, Nussenblatt RB, et al. Association of interleukin 10 in the vitreous and cerebrospinal fluid and primary central nervous system lymphoma. Arch Ophthalmol. 1997;115(9):1157–60.
8. Commins DL. Pathology of primary central nervous system lymphoma. Neurosurg Focus. 2006;21(5):E2.
9. Salomão DR, Pulido JS, Johnston PB, Canal-Fontcuberta I, Feldman AL. Vitreoretinal presentation of secondary large B-cell lymphoma in patients with systemic lymphoma. JAMA Ophthalmol. 2013;131(9):1151–8.
10. Grimm SA, McCannel CA, Omuro AMP, Ferreri AJM, Blay J-Y, Neuwelt EA, et al. Primary CNS lymphoma with intraocular involvement: International PCNSL Collaborative Group Report. Neurology. 2008;71(17):1355–60.
11. Alizadeh AA, Eisen MB, Davis RE, Ma C, Lossos IS, Rosenwald A, et al. Distinct types of diffuse large B-cell lymphoma identified by gene expression profiling. Nature. 2000;403(6769):503–11.
12. Choi WWL, Weisenburger DD, Greiner TC, Piris MA, Banham AH, Delabie J, et al. A new immunostain algorithm classifies diffuse large B-cell lymphoma into molecular subtypes with high accuracy. Clin Cancer Res. 2009;15(17):5494–502.
13. Ryan SJ, Zimmerman LE, King FM. Reactive lymphoid hyperplasia. An unusual form of intraocular pseudotumor. Trans Am Acad Ophthalmol Otolaryngol. 1972;76(3):652–71.
14. Grossniklaus HE, Martin DF, Avery R, Shields JA, Shields CL, Kuo IC, et al. Uveal lymphoid infiltration. Report of four cases and clinicopathologic review. Ophthalmology. 1998;105(7):1265–73.
15. Knowles DM, Jakobiec FA, McNally L, Burke JS. Lymphoid hyperplasia and malignant lymphoma occurring in the ocular adnexa (orbit, conjunctiva, and eyelids): a prospective multiparametric analysis of 108 cases during 1977 to 1987. Hum Pathol. 1990;21(9):959–73.
16. Coupland SE, Damato B. Understanding intraocular lymphomas. Clin Exp Ophthalmol. 2008;36(6):564–78.
17. Cook JR, Isaacson PG, Chott A, Nakamura S, Muller-Hermelink HK, Harris NL, et al. Extranodal marginal zone lymphoma of mucosa-associated lymphoid tissue (MALT lymphoma). WHO classification of tumours of haematopoietic and lymphoid tissues. 4th ed. Lyon: IARC; 2016. p. 259–65.
18. Mashayekhi A, Shields CL, Shields JA. Iris involvement by lymphoma: a review of 13 cases. Clin Exp Ophthalmol. 2013;41(1):19–26.
19. Velez G, de Smet MD, Whitcup SM, Robinson M, Nussenblatt RB, Chan CC. Iris involvement in primary intraocular lymphoma: report of two cases and review of the literature. Surv Ophthalmol. 2000;44(6):518–26.
20. Ferry JA, Fung CY, Zukerberg L, Lucarelli MJ, Hasserjian RP, Preffer FI, et al. Lymphoma of the ocular adnexa: a study of 353 cases. Am J Surg Pathol. 2007;31(2):170–84.
21. White WL, Ferry JA, Harris NL, Grove AS. Ocular adnexal lymphoma. A clinicopathologic study with identification of lymphomas of mucosa-associated lymphoid tissue type. Ophthalmology. 1995;102(12):1994–2006.
22. Harris NL, Isaacson PG. What are the criteria for distinguishing MALT from non-MALT lymphoma at

extranodal sites? Am J Clin Pathol. 1999;111(1 Suppl 1):S126–32.
23. Ruiz A, Reischl U, Swerdlow SH, Hartke M, Streubel B, Procop G, et al. Extranodal marginal zone B-cell lymphomas of the ocular adnexa: multiparameter analysis of 34 cases including interphase molecular cytogenetics and PCR for Chlamydia psittaci. Am J Surg Pathol. 2007;31(5):792–802.
24. Coupland SE, Krause L, Delecluse HJ, Anagnostopoulos I, Foss HD, Hummel M, et al. Lymphoproliferative lesions of the ocular adnexa. Analysis of 112 cases. Ophthalmology. 1998;105(8):1430–41.
25. Wang Z, Cook JR. IRTA1 and MNDA expression in marginal zone lymphoma: utility in differential diagnosis and implications for classification. Am J Clin Pathol. 2019;151(3):337–43.
26. Evans PS, Pott C, Groenen PJTA, Salles G, Davi F, Berger F, et al. Significantly improved PCR-based clonality testing in B-cell malignancies by use of multiple immunoglobulin gene targets. Report of the BIOMED-2 Concerted Action BHM4-CT98-3936. Leukemia. 2007;21(2):207–14.
27. Guo L, Wang Z, Anderson CM, Doolittle E, Kernag S, Cotta CV, et al. Ultrasensitive automated RNA in situ hybridization for kappa and lambda light chain mRNA detects B-cell clonality in tissue biopsies with performance comparable or superior to flow cytometry. Mod Pathol. 2018;31(3):385–94.
28. Remstein ED, Dogan A, Einerson RR, Paternoster SF, Fink SR, Law M, et al. The incidence and anatomic site specificity of chromosomal translocations in primary extranodal marginal zone B-cell lymphoma of mucosa-associated lymphoid tissue (MALT lymphoma) in North America. Am J Surg Pathol. 2006;30(12):1546–53.
29. Streubel B, Lamprecht A, Dierlamm J, Cerroni L, Stolte M, Ott G, et al. T(14;18)(q32;q21) involving IGH and MALT1 is a frequent chromosomal aberration in MALT lymphoma. Blood. 2003;101(6):2335–9.
30. Akagi T, Motegi M, Tamura A, Suzuki R, Hosokawa Y, Suzuki H, et al. A novel gene, MALT1 at 18q21, is involved in t(11;18) (q21;q21) found in low-grade B-cell lymphoma of mucosa-associated lymphoid tissue. Oncogene. 1999;18(42):5785–94.
31. Willis TG, Jadayel DM, Du MQ, Peng H, Perry AR, Abdul-Rauf M, et al. Bcl10 is involved in t(1;14) (p22;q32) of MALT B cell lymphoma and mutated in multiple tumor types. Cell. 1999;96(1):35–45.
32. Chanudet E, Huang Y, Ichimura K, Dong G, Hamoudi RA, Radford J, et al. A20 is targeted by promoter methylation, deletion and inactivating mutation in MALT lymphoma. Leukemia. 2010;24(2):483–7.
33. Ferreri AJM, Dolcetti R, Dognini GP, Malabarba L, Vicari N, Pasini E, et al. Chlamydophila psittaci is viable and infectious in the conjunctiva and peripheral blood of patients with ocular adnexal lymphoma: results of a single-center prospective case–control study. Int J Cancer. 2008;123(5):1089–93.
34. Decaudin D, Dolcetti R, de Cremoux P, Ponzoni M, Vincent-Salomon A, Doglioni C, et al. Variable association between Chlamydophila psittaci infection and ocular adnexal lymphomas: methodological biases or true geographical variations? Anti-Cancer Drugs. 2008;19(8):761–5.
35. Sehn LH, Salles G. Diffuse large B-cell lymphoma. N Engl J Med. 2021;384(9):842–58.
36. Khanlari M, Chapman JR. Follicular lymphoma: updates for pathologists. J Pathol Transl Med. 2022;56(1):1–15.
37. Knudsen MKH, Rasmussen PK, Coupland SE, Esmaeli B, Finger PT, Graue GF, et al. Clinicopathological features of ocular adnexal mantle-cell lymphoma in an international multicenter cohort. JAMA Ophthalmol. 2017;135(12):1367–74.
38. Moslehi R, Devesa SS, Schairer C, Fraumeni JF. Rapidly increasing incidence of ocular non-Hodgkin lymphoma. J Natl Cancer Inst. 2006;98(13):936–9.

4 Mutational Profile of Ocular Lymphoma

Christopher Seungkyu Lee

Introduction

Classification system of lymphoma has evolved with heated debates since Thomas Hodgkin first described lymphomas in 1832 [1]. Worldwide consensus has only been made in the last two decades or so when the International Lymphoma Study Group published REAL classification in 1994 [2], which has led to the development of modern WHO classification in 2001 [3]. A multi-parameter approach is used in the current consensus classification, which takes into account all available information including clinical features, morphology, immunophenotype, and genetics. The relative importance of each feature differs according to the disease, but genetic abnormalities are gaining importance in disease definition, thanks to recent progress in our understanding of lymphoma genetics. In the following chapter, the genetic abnormalities and molecular profiles of ocular lymphomas will be reviewed.

C. S. Lee (✉)
Department of Ophthalmology, The Institute of Vision Research, Yonsei University College of Medicine, Seoul, Korea
e-mail: sklee219@yuhs.ac

Definition of Ocular Lymphoma

Ocular lymphomas can be divided into intraocular lymphomas involving vitreous, retina, and uvea, and ocular adnexal lymphomas involving orbit, conjunctiva, lacrimal gland, and eyelid. The most common type of intraocular lymphomas is the vitreoretinal lymphoma, usually diffuse large B-cell lymphoma (DLBCL) of high-grade malignancy with frequent involvement of the central nervous system (CNS) [4]. PCNSL-O is the preferred term to emphasize that it is an ocular variant or subset of primary CNS lymphoma (PCNSL). Uveal lymphoma is an extremely rare type of intraocular lymphomas and is usually extranodal marginal zone B-cell lymphoma (EMZL) of low-grade malignancy [5]. EMZL is also the most common subtype of ocular adnexal lymphomas, accounting for about two-third of cases [6].

Mutational Profile of Intraocular Lymphoma

PCNSL-O is considered a variant of primary CNS lymphoma. PCNSL-O is the preferred term to emphasize that it is an ocular variant or subset of primary CNS lymphoma (PCNSL). About 50–80% of PCNSL-O patients develop CNS disease within several years [7, 8]. Conversely, about 15–25% of primary CNS lymphoma

V. R. Raval et al. (eds.), *Ocular and Adnexal Lymphoma*, Essentials in Ophthalmology,
https://doi.org/10.1007/978-3-031-24595-4_4

Table 4.1 Mutational profile in vitreoretinal lymphoma

Altered genes	Frequency (%)	Possible functions	References
MYD88	57.1–100	NF-κB pathway	[24, 25, 27, 28, 31–33, 37, 38]
CD79B	22.2–55	NF-κB pathway	[24, 28, 37, 39]
IGLL5	52–88.9	B-cell development	[28, 37]
PIM1	71–88.9	Serine/threonine kinase	[28, 37]
TBL1XR1	48	Transcription regulation	[34]
ETV6	45	Transcription regulation	[34]
CDKN2A	66.7–100	Tumor suppressor	[28, 37, 38]
BTG2	77.8	Tumor suppressor	[28]
BTG1	55.6	Tumor suppressor	[28]
PTEN	25	Tumor suppressor	[38]

B-cell receptor signaling and NF-κB activation [39]. Biallelic or monoallelic deletion of the tumor suppressor CDKN2A is also a frequent finding in PCNSL-O ranging from 66.7% to 100% [28, 37, 38].

Primary uveal lymphomas are typically EMZL [5]. The genotype or mutational profile has not been studied much due to rarity of the disease, but their morphological and immunophenotypical features seem to be similar to EMZL of other locations [40]. Chromosomal translocation t(11;18)(q21;1q21) (BIRC3/MALT1) has been observed in one study [40].

Mutational Profile of Ocular Adnexal Lymphoma

EMZL is the most common subtype of ocular adnexal lymphoma [6]. When involving an overlying epithelium such as the conjunctiva or acini of the lacrimal gland, the term "mucosa-associated lymphatic tissue (MALT)" lymphomas are often used instead. But many studies also use the term MALT lymphomas for diseases involving orbital compartment where no epithelium is present. In this chapter, the term EMZL will be used, which would be a more accurate term referring to lymphomas arising in all parts of ocular adnexa. Follicular lymphoma (10–15%), DLBCL (8–13%), and rare mantle cell lymphoma (1–5%) constitute the rest [6, 41]. EMZL and follicular lymphoma generally show better prognosis than DLBCL and mantle cell lymphoma.

Ocular adnexal MALT lymphomas derive from post-germinal center B cells [41]. Chronic infections by *Chlamydia psittaci* have been linked to the pathogenesis of ocular adnexal MALT lymphomas in some geographical regions [42]. Various chromosomal translocations including (1;14)(p22;q32)(BCL10/IgH), t(14;18)(q32;p21)(IgH/MALT1), t(11;18)(q21;1q21)(BIRC3/MALT1), and t(3;14)(p14;q32)(FOXP1/IgH) are frequently seen in EMZL of other locations including lung and stomach, but they are rarely or not detected in ocular adnexal EMZL [43, 44]. In contrast, mutation or deletion in TNFAIP3, a NF-κB negative regulator, is frequently seen in ocular adnexal EMZL, but not commonly seen in EMZL of other sites [43–45]. Constitute activation of NF-κB signaling pathway is a hallmark finding of ocular adnexal EMZL and TNFAIP3 appears to be the major driver gene in terms of frequency and known functional aspects [43, 44, 46, 47]. Mutations of TNFAIP3, along with other frequently mutated genes involved in NF-κB pathway including, MYD88, BCL10, and CD79B may be collectively involved in oncogenesis of ocular adnexal EMZL via NF-κB signaling pathway [43, 48]. Other frequently mutated genes by whole exome or whole genome sequencing include TBL1XR1 and CREBBP [43, 44]. TBL1XR1 can activate transcription factors such as NF-κB and JUN and promote tumor cell survival [44]. CREBBP is an epigenetic regulator, encoding a histone/protein acetyltransferase. Mutations were also reported in other epigenetic regulators KMT2D and KMT2C in ocular adnexal EMZL [43, 46]. These findings suggest that epigenetic dysregulation is involved in pathogenesis of ocular adnexal EMZL in addition to activated NF-κB pathway [43]. Other frequently mutated genes reported include NOTCH1, NOTCH2, TET2, LRP1B, JAK3, LRP1B, COL12A1, COL1A2, DOCK8, TP53, PRDM1 (Table 4.2) [44, 46, 48].

Molecular studies in ocular adnexal follicular lymphomas and DLBCL are few due to their rarity. Their molecular alterations may follow genotypic patterns of systemic follicular lymphomas and DLBCL. MYD88 mutation is more frequently seen in ocular adnexal DLBCL than in ocular adnexal EMZL [49]. Mutations in epigenetic modulators, EZH2 and ARID1A were both common in ocular adnexal DLBCL and ocular adnexal follicular lymphoma in one study [49]. Mutations in histone methyltransferases KMT2B in ocular adnexal follicular lymphoma and KMT3B in ocular adnexal DLBCL were also seen [49]. Other frequently seen mutations include CDKN2A, PTEN, ATM, NF1, NRAS in ocular adnexal DLBCL, and HRAS in follicular lymphoma [49].

Table 4.2 Mutational profile of ocular adnexal extranodal marginal zone B-cell lymphoma

Altered genes	Frequency (%)	Functions	References
TNFAIP3	27–54	NF-κB pathway	[43, 44, 46–48]
MYD88	4–25	NF-κB pathway	[43, 46–49]
BCL10	4–6	NF-κB pathway	[43, 48]
CD79B	2–4	NF-κB pathway	[43, 48]
TBL1XR1	6–19	Transcription regulation	[43, 44, 47]
CREBBP	13–25	Epigenetic regulation	[43, 44, 46]
KMT2D	6–22	Epigenetic regulation	[43, 46, 48]
KMT2C	25	Epigenetic regulation	[46]
TET2	15	Epigenetic regulation	[46]
NOTCH1	2–8	B-cell differentiation	[43, 47–49]
NOTCH2	8–15	B-cell differentiation	[46, 48]
DOCK8	6	B-cell differentiation	[44]
JAK3	11	JAK/STAT pathway	[44]
COL12A1	7	Cell adhesion	[44]
COL1A2	6	Cell adhesion	[44]
LRP1B	6–25	Tumor suppressor	[43, 46]
TP53	8	Tumor suppressor	[48]

Conclusions

Lymphoma is one of the most heterogeneous groups of malignancies with complicated classification systems. The heterogeneity in lymphoma owes primarily to the complex features of development and differentiation of B-cell and T-cell lymphocytes. Recent progress in our understanding of pathogenesis and clinical course of lymphomas was made with GEP studies that even changed how we classify lymphomas (e.g. GCB and ABC subtypes in DLBCL). Mutational profiles of ocular lymphomas seemed to be different from lymphomas of the "same subtype" occurring at other sites. Mutational profile of vitreoretinal DLBCL is characterized by the high, if not the highest, frequency of MYD88 mutation among DLBCLs, possibly in association with ocular immune privilege and it does not seem to simply fit into either GCB and ABC subtypes. Chromosomal translocations are frequently seen in EMZL of other sites, but not in ocular adnexal EMZL. By contrast, somatic mutations, especially TNFAIP3 mutation, are frequently detected in ocular adnexal EMZL, while they are less commonly seen in EMZL of other sites. Further genetic studies are warranted, especially in other rare subtypes of ocular lymphomas, that will advance our understanding and management of ocular lymphomas.

References

1. Hodgkin T. On some morbid appearances of the absorbent glands and spleen. Med Chir Trans. 1832;17:68–114.
2. Harris NL, Jaffe ES, Stein H, Banks PM, Chan JK, Cleary ML, et al. A revised European-American classification of lymphoid neoplasms: a proposal from the International Lymphoma Study Group. Blood. 1994;84(5):1361–92.

3. Jaffe E, Harris N, Stein H, Vardiman JW. Pathology and genetics of tumours of haematopoetic and lymphoid tissues – World Health Organization Classification of Tumours. 3rd ed. Lyon: IARC Press; 2001.
4. Chan CC. Primary intraocular lymphoma: clinical features, diagnosis, and treatment. Clin Lymphoma. 2003;4(1):30–1.
5. Coupland SE, Foss HD, Hidayat AA, Cockerham GC, Hummel M, Stein H. Extranodal marginal zone B cell lymphomas of the uvea: an analysis of 13 cases. J Pathol. 2002;197(3):333–40.
6. Coupland SE, Krause L, Delecluse HJ, Anagnostopoulos I, Foss HD, Hummel M, et al. Lymphoproliferative lesions of the ocular adnexa. Analysis of 112 cases. Ophthalmology. 1998;105(8):1430–41.
7. Peterson K, Gordon KB, Heinemann MH, DeAngelis LM. The clinical spectrum of ocular lymphoma. Cancer. 1993;72(3):843–9.
8. Akpek EK, Ahmed I, Hochberg FH, Soheilian M, Dryja TP, Jakobiec FA, et al. Intraocular-central nervous system lymphoma: clinical features, diagnosis, and outcomes. Ophthalmology. 1999;106(9):1805–10.
9. Rockwood EJ, Zakov ZN, Bay JW. Combined malignant lymphoma of the eye and CNS (reticulum-cell sarcoma). Report of three cases. J Neurosurg. 1984;61(2):369–74.
10. Rothova A, Ooijman F, Kerkhoff F, Van Der Lelij A, Lokhorst HM. Uveitis masquerade syndromes. Ophthalmology. 2001;108(2):386–99.
11. Nussenblatt RB, Chan CC, Wilson WH, Hochman J, Gottesman M, CNS, et al. International Central Nervous System and Ocular Lymphoma Workshop: recommendations for the future. Ocul Immunol Inflamm. 2006;14(3):139–44.
12. Reichstein D. Primary vitreoretinal lymphoma: an update on pathogenesis, diagnosis and treatment. Curr Opin Ophthalmol. 2016;27(3):177–84.
13. Lee J, Kim SW, Kim H, Lee CS, Kim M, Lee SC. Differential diagnosis for vitreoretinal lymphoma with vitreoretinal findings, immunoglobulin clonality tests, and interleukin levels. Retina. 2019;39(6):1165–76.
14. Chan CC. Molecular pathology of primary intraocular lymphoma. Trans Am Ophthalmol Soc. 2003;101:275–92.
15. Kohno T, Uchida H, Inomata H, Fukushima S, Takeshita M, Kikuchi M. Ocular manifestations of adult T-cell leukemia/lymphoma. A clinicopathologic study. Ophthalmology. 1993;100(12):1794–9.
16. Whitcup SM, de Smet MD, Rubin BI, Palestine AG, Martin DF, Burnier M Jr, et al. Intraocular lymphoma. Clin Histopathol Diagn Ophthalmol. 1993;100(9):1399–406.
17. Siegel RL, Miller KD, Jemal A. Cancer statistics, 2015. CA Cancer J Clin. 2015;65(1):5–29.
18. Alizadeh AA, Eisen MB, Davis RE, Ma C, Lossos IS, Rosenwald A, et al. Distinct types of diffuse large B-cell lymphoma identified by gene expression profiling. Nature. 2000;403(6769):503–11.
19. Staudt LM, Dave S. The biology of human lymphoid malignancies revealed by gene expression profiling. Adv Immunol. 2005;87:163–208.
20. Lenz G, Wright GW, Emre NC, Kohlhammer H, Dave SS, Davis RE, et al. Molecular subtypes of diffuse large B-cell lymphoma arise by distinct genetic pathways. Proc Natl Acad Sci U S A. 2008;105(36):13520–5.
21. Li S, Young KH, Medeiros LJ. Diffuse large B-cell lymphoma. Pathology. 2018;50(1):74–87.
22. Rosenwald A, Wright G, Leroy K, Yu X, Gaulard P, Gascoyne RD, et al. Molecular diagnosis of primary mediastinal B cell lymphoma identifies a clinically favorable subgroup of diffuse large B cell lymphoma related to Hodgkin lymphoma. J Exp Med. 2003;198(6):851–62.
23. Wallace DJ, Shen D, Reed GF, Miyanaga M, Mochizuki M, Sen HN, et al. Detection of the bcl-2 t(14;18) translocation and proto-oncogene expression in primary intraocular lymphoma. Invest Ophthalmol Vis Sci. 2006;47(7):2750–6.
24. Arai A, Takase H, Yoshimori M, Yamamoto K, Mochizuki M, Miura O. Gene expression profiling of primary vitreoretinal lymphoma. Cancer Sci. 2020;111(4):1417–21.
25. Bonzheim I, Giese S, Deuter C, Susskind D, Zierhut M, Waizel M, et al. High frequency of MYD88 mutations in vitreoretinal B-cell lymphoma: a valuable tool to improve diagnostic yield of vitreous aspirates. Blood. 2015;126(1):76–9.
26. Nakamura T, Tateishi K, Niwa T, Matsushita Y, Tamura K, Kinoshita M, et al. Recurrent mutations of CD79B and MYD88 are the hallmark of primary central nervous system lymphomas. Neuropathol Appl Neurobiol. 2016;42(3):279–90.
27. Raja H, Salomao DR, Viswanatha DS, Pulido JS. Prevalence of Myd88 L265p mutation in histologically proven, diffuse large B-cell vitreoretinal lymphoma. Retina. 2016;36(3):624–8.
28. Lee J, Kim B, Lee H, Park H, Ho Byeon S, Choi JR, et al. Whole exome sequencing identifies mutational signatures of vitreoretinal lymphoma. Haematologica. 2020;105(9):e458–60.
29. Schmitz R, Wright GW, Huang DW, Johnson CA, Phelan JD, Wang JQ, et al. Genetics and pathogenesis of diffuse large B-cell lymphoma. N Engl J Med. 2018;378(15):1396–407.
30. Lee JH, Jeong H, Choi JW, Oh H, Kim YS. Clinicopathologic significance of MYD88 L265P mutation in diffuse large B-cell lymphoma: a meta-analysis. Sci Rep. 2017;7(1):1785.
31. Pulido JS, Salomao DR, Frederick LA, Viswanatha DS. MyD-88 L265P mutations are present in some cases of vitreoretinal lymphoma. Retina. 2015;35(4):624–7.
32. Miserocchi E, Ferreri AJM, Giuffre C, Cangi MG, Francaviglia I, Calimeri T, et al. Myd88 L265p mutation detection in the aqueous humor of patients with vitreoretinal lymphoma. Retina. 2019;39(4):679–84.

33. Hiemcke-Jiwa LS, Ten Dam-van Loon NH, Leguit RJ, Nierkens S, Ossewaarde-van Norel J, de Boer JH, et al. Potential diagnosis of vitreoretinal lymphoma by detection of MYD88 mutation in aqueous humor with ultrasensitive droplet digital polymerase chain reaction. JAMA Ophthalmol. 2018;136(10):1098–104.
34. Choi S, Shin S, Lee ST, Lee J, Lee JS, Kim B, et al. Serial detection of MYD88 L265P mutation in the aqueous humor of a patient with vitreoretinal lymphoma for disease monitoring. Ocul Immunol Inflamm. 2021;29(3):485–9.
35. Jeelall YS, Horikawa K. Oncogenic MYD88 mutation drives Toll pathway to lymphoma. Immunol Cell Biol. 2011;89(6):659–60.
36. Wright GW, Huang DW, Phelan JD, Coulibaly ZA, Roulland S, Young RM, et al. A probabilistic classification tool for genetic subtypes of diffuse large B cell lymphoma with therapeutic implications. Cancer Cell. 2020;37(4):551–68 e14.
37. Bonzheim I, Sander P, Salmeron-Villalobos J, Susskind D, Szurman P, Gekeler F, et al. The molecular hallmarks of primary and secondary vitreoretinal lymphoma. Blood Adv. 2021;6:1598.
38. Cani AK, Hovelson DH, Demirci H, Johnson MW, Tomlins SA, Rao RC. Next generation sequencing of vitreoretinal lymphomas from small-volume intraocular liquid biopsies: new routes to targeted therapies. Oncotarget. 2017;8(5):7989–98.
39. Yonese I, Takase H, Yoshimori M, Onozawa E, Tsuzura A, Miki T, et al. CD79B mutations in primary vitreoretinal lymphoma: diagnostic and prognostic potential. Eur J Haematol. 2019;102(2):191–6.
40. Coupland SE, Damato B. Understanding intraocular lymphomas. Clin Exp Ophthalmol. 2008;36(6):564–78.
41. McKelvie PA. Ocular adnexal lymphomas: a review. Adv Anat Pathol. 2010;17(4):251–61.
42. Chanudet E, Zhou Y, Bacon CM, Wotherspoon AC, Muller-Hermelink HK, Adam P, et al. Chlamydia psittaci is variably associated with ocular adnexal MALT lymphoma in different geographical regions. J Pathol. 2006;209(3):344–51.
43. Jung H, Yoo HY, Lee SH, Shin S, Kim SC, Lee S, et al. The mutational landscape of ocular marginal zone lymphoma identifies frequent alterations in TNFAIP3 followed by mutations in TBL1XR1 and CREBBP. Oncotarget. 2017;8(10):17038–49.
44. Johansson P, Klein-Hitpass L, Budeus B, Kuhn M, Lauber C, Seifert M, et al. Identifying genetic lesions in ocular adnexal extranodal marginal zone lymphomas of the MALT subtype by whole genome, whole exome and targeted sequencing. Cancers. 2020;12(4):986.
45. Honma K, Tsuzuki S, Nakagawa M, Tagawa H, Nakamura S, Morishima Y, et al. TNFAIP3/A20 functions as a novel tumor suppressor gene in several subtypes of non-Hodgkin lymphomas. Blood. 2009;114(12):2467–75.
46. Cascione L, Rinaldi A, Bruscaggin A, Tarantelli C, Arribas AJ, Kwee I, et al. Novel insights into the genetics and epigenetics of MALT lymphoma unveiled by next generation sequencing analyses. Haematologica. 2019;104(12):e558–e61.
47. Moody S, Thompson JS, Chuang SS, Liu H, Raderer M, Vassiliou G, et al. Novel GPR34 and CCR6 mutation and distinct genetic profiles in MALT lymphomas of different sites. Haematologica. 2018;103(8):1329–36.
48. Johansson P, Klein-Hitpass L, Grabellus F, Arnold G, Klapper W, Pfortner R, et al. Recurrent mutations in NF-kappaB pathway components, KMT2D, and NOTCH1/2 in ocular adnexal MALT-type marginal zone lymphomas. Oncotarget. 2016;7(38):62627–39.
49. Cani AK, Soliman M, Hovelson DH, Liu CJ, McDaniel AS, Haller MJ, et al. Comprehensive genomic profiling of orbital and ocular adnexal lymphomas identifies frequent alterations in MYD88 and chromatin modifiers: new routes to targeted therapies. Mod Pathol. 2016;29(7):685–97.

Ocular Adnexal Lymphoma: Clinical Presentation and Imaging Studies

5

Kavya Madhuri Bejjanki and Swathi Kaliki

Introduction

Primary ocular adnexal lymphoma (OAL) is defined as the tumor arising from conjunctiva, orbit including extraocular muscles and lacrimal gland, eyelids, and lacrimal sac. When the tumor arises from the extraorbital site and spreads to the ocular adnexa, it is termed secondary ocular adnexal lymphoma (5%) [1]. Lymphomas are the most common malignant tumors in ocular adnexa. The overall incidence rate of primary OAL is 1–2% of all non-Hodgkin's lymphomas (NHL) and 5–10% of all extranodal NHL with increasing trend noted in the recent times [2, 3].

Classification

Ann Arbor Staging System [4]

This is the landmark classification system for staging both Hodgkin and non-Hodgkin lymphoma.

- **Stage I:** Involvement of a single lymph node region or of a single extralymphatic organ or site
- **Stage II:** Involvement of two or more lymph node regions on the same side of the diaphragm or localized involvement of an extralymphatic organ or site
- **Stage III:** Involvement of lymph node regions or structures on both sides of the diaphragm
- **Stage IV:** Diffuse or disseminated involvement of one or more extralymphatic organs, or either:
  - Isolated extralymphatic organ involvement without adjacent regional lymph node involvement, but with disease in distant sites
  - Involvement of the liver, bone marrow, pleura, or cerebrospinal fluid

Additional substaging variables include:

- **A:** Asymptomatic
- **B:** Presence of B symptoms (including fever, night sweats, and weight loss of ≥10% of body weight over 6 months)
- **E**: Involvement of a single, extranodal site, contiguous or proximal to a known nodal site (stages I–III only; additional extranodal involvement is stage IV)
- **S**: Splenic involvement
- **X:** Bulky Nodal Disease: nodal mass >1/3 of intrathoracic diameter or 10 cm in dimension [4].

K. M. Bejjanki
Hima Bindu Yalamanchili Centre for Eye Cancer, Operation Eyesight Universal Institute for Eye Cancer, L V Prasad Eye Institute, Vijayawada, India

S. Kaliki (✉)
The Operation Eyesight Universal Institute for Eye Cancer, L V Prasad Eye Institute, Hyderabad, India

V. R. Raval et al. (eds.), *Ocular and Adnexal Lymphoma*, Essentials in Ophthalmology,
https://doi.org/10.1007/978-3-031-24595-4_5

American Joint Committee on Cancer (AJCC) Classification [5]

As Ann Arbor staging system has its own limitations in staging the OAL accurately, AJCC classification was introduced based on the location of the primary tumor (T), lymph node involvement (L), and distant metastasis (M). It is useful in predicting the long-term survival of the patient by describing the laterality of the disease along with lymph node and distant metastasis in the initial presentation of the OAL [5]. *AJCC classification is currently in its eighth edition and the classification is as follows.*

Primary Tumor (T)

- TX: Lymphoma extent not specified
- T0: No evidence of lymphoma
- T1: Lymphoma involving only conjunctiva without eyelid or orbital involvement
- T2: Lymphoma with orbital involvement with/without conjunctival involvement
- T3: Lymphoma with preseptal eyelid involvement with/without orbital and/or conjunctival involvement
- T4: Orbital adnexal lymphoma and extraorbital lymphoma extending beyond orbit to adjacent structures, such as bone, paranasal sinuses, and brain

Lymph Node Involvement (N)

- NX: Involvement of lymph nodes not assessed
- N0: No evidence of lymph node involvement
- N1: Involvement of regional lymph nodes draining the ocular adnexal structures and superior to the mediastinum (preauricular, parotid, submandibular, and cervical lymph nodes)
- N1a: Involvement of single lymph node region above the mediastinum
- N1b: Involvement of two or more lymph node regions above the mediastinum
- N2: Involvement of lymph node regions of the mediastinum
- N3: Diffuse involvement of peripheral and central lymph node regions

Distal Metastasis (M)

- M0: No evidence of involvement of other extranodal sites
- M1: Lymphomatous involvement in other organs
- M1a: Noncontiguous involvement of tissues or organs outside the ocular adnexa (e.g., parotid gland, submandibular gland, lung, liver, spleen, kidney, breast)
- M1b: Lymphomatous involvement of the bone marrow
- M1c: Both M1 and M1b involvement [6]

Lugano Classification [7]

Based on the assessment of response by imaging (PET-CT), this classification system was proposed.

Limited

- **Stage I:** One node or group of adjacent nodes
  - **Stage IE**: Single extralymphatic site in the absence of nodal involvement
- **Stage II:** Two or more nodal groups, same side of diaphragm
  - **Stage IIE**: Contiguous extralymphatic extension from a nodal site with or without involvement of other lymph node regions on the same side of the diaphragm.

Advanced

- **Stage III:** Nodes on both sides of the diaphragm; nodes above the diaphragm with spleen involvement
  - **Stage III (1):** Involvement of the spleen or splenic, hilar, coeliac, or portal nodes
  - **Stage III (2):** Involvement of the para-aortic, iliac, inguinal, or mesenteric nodes
- **Stage IV:** Diffuse or disseminated involvement of one or more extranodal organs or tissue beyond that designated E, with or without associated lymph node involvement

1. All cases to indicate the absence (**A**) or presence (**B**) of systemic symptoms (fever/night sweats/unexplained weight loss)

2. Designation of (**E**) refers to extranodal contiguous extension that can still be encompassed within irradiation field appropriate for nodal disease of the same anatomic extent (if more extensive than that, label as **IV**)
3. Designation of (bulky) if a single nodal mass >10 cm or >1/3 of transthoracic diameter [7].

LYRIC (Lymphoma Response to Immunomodulatory Therapy Criteria) Classification [8]

This classification system is adapted from the Lugano classification and based on the response to immunomodulators, "Indeterminate response" was added in addition.

Indeterminate Response (IR)

- IR (1): ≥50% increase in overall tumor burden (sum of the product of the perpendicular diameters (SPD) of up to six target measurable nodes and extranodal sites) occurred in the first 12 weeks of therapy and without clinical deterioration
- IR (2): New lesions or ≥50% increase of existing lesion(s) without a ≥50% increase of overall tumor burden at any time during treatment.
- IR (3): Increased FDG uptake of one or more lesions without any increase in size or number of those lesions.

If two patterns of IR are present at the same time, priority should be given to IR (1) or (2) over IR (3).

After an IR, a biopsy or subsequent imaging within 12 weeks is recommended to confirm true progressive disease versus a flare or pseudoprogression [8].

Conjunctival OAL

1. Incidence: 30–40% of OALs [9].

   Age and Gender: Conjunctival OAL typically affects elderly population between fifth and seventh decade with predominant female preponderance [10].

   Distribution: Conjunctival OALs are predominantly EMZL type of B-cell lymphomas [11].
2. Symptoms: Most of the time, the presentation is of insidious onset and slowly progressive with minimal symptoms. The complaints are widely variable ranging from non-specific eye redness, irritation, watering to prominent conjunctival mass, drooping of eyelid and double vision, depending upon the location and extent of the lesion.

   Signs: It is characterized by "Salmon color patch," a subconjunctival pink fleshy mass. It is commonly located in the bulbar conjunctiva and sometimes in the forniceal and palpebral conjunctiva. It is important to rule out associated eyelid and orbital components by detailed periocular examination [12].
3. Differential Diagnoses: Conjunctival amelanotic melanoma, subconjunctival fat prolapse, myxomatous lesions, leiomyosarcomas, and juvenile xanthogranuloma.

Orbital OAL

1. Incidence: 50–60% of OALs [13].

   Age and Gender: Though the age distribution varies depending on the subtype, orbital lymphomas are commonly seen in elderly population. Though female preponderance was shown in some studies, there is no gender predilection as such [14].

   Distribution: Majority of the subtypes of orbital OALs are of B-cell in origin (>95%), whereas T-cell and NKT-cell subtypes are less frequently seen (<5%) [15].

   Extranodal marginal zone lymphoma (EMZL), also termed MALT lymphoma, is the most common B-cell lymphoma (>50%). Its course is indolent in nature even in extensive disease. Systemic association is seen in nearly 25% with relapse rate seen in one-third of the patients at extraocular sites. But, it has an excellent prognosis with a 5-year progression free survival rate of 71% and overall survival rate of about 75%. MALT 1 and IGH gene loci are helpful in predicting the relapse rate of orbital EMZL [16, 17].

Other common B-cell lymphomas are diffuse large B-cell lymphoma (DLBCL), follicular lymphoma (FL), mantle cell lymphoma (MCL) with the incidence rates of 23%, 9%, 5% and the overall survival rates of 36%, 60%, <40%, respectively.

2. Symptoms and Signs: The clinical presentation depends on the involvement of the orbital quadrant and the extent of the lesion. It is insidious in onset, painless, slowly progressive with patients often complaining of protrusion of eyes, periocular fullness and presents with proptosis, dystopia, ptosis, palpable orbital mass, diplopia, motility restriction, and optic nerve compression [18].

   Orbital OALs are most commonly located in the superior quadrant of orbit extending intraconally (8%), extraconally (72%) or both (11%). Due to the mass effect of the lesion, the patient develops gradually progressive proptosis and displacement of the eyeball [19].

   If the tumor is infiltrating the extraocular muscles (9%), it results in diplopia, strabismus, and motility restriction. Recti muscles (>70%) are more commonly involved than oblique muscles (<20%). Superior rectus followed by inferior and lateral rectus are the commonly infiltrated extraocular muscles [20].

   Atypical Presentation: Rarely, atypical presentations like painful proptosis, inflammation mimicking orbital cellulitis, defective vision are associated with highly malignant and rapidly progressive B-cell lymphoma subtypes like DLBCL, MCL, and HIV related lymphoma. Orbital inflammation results from direct invasion of orbital soft tissues by tumor cells or by secondary invasion from paranasal sinuses. The patient presents with periorbital swelling, conjunctival congestion, and chemosis in the initial visit masquerading orbital cellulitis or other orbital inflammatory diseases. These signs hamper early diagnosis and management of these patients. In spite of medical management, if the orbital cellulitis progresses or worsens, malignancy should be considered as an alternative diagnosis. Visual impairment is seen when the tumor enlarges in size in the apical region of orbit causing compression or infiltration of the optic nerve [21, 22].

   T-cell and natural killer T-cell lymphomas are also commonly located in the extraconal space. When compared to B-cell lymphomas, T-cell and NKT-cell lymphomas have higher incidence of extraocular muscle involvement [23–27].

3. Differential Diagnoses: Infectious orbital diseases, inflammatory conditions such as non-specific inflammatory disease, reactive lymphoid hyperplasias, orbital leukemic infiltrates, vascular tumors, and orbital metastasis.

Lacrimal Gland Lymphoma

1. Incidence: 7–26% of OALs.

   Age and Gender: It is predominantly seen in elderly population with female preponderance [25].

   Distribution: Lacrimal gland lymphomas comprise 51% of orbital B-cell lymphomas and 24% of T-cell lymphomas. Though EMZL is the most common subtype of B-cell lymphomas, the incidence is less frequent when compared to the orbital OALs, whereas follicular lymphoma is more commonly seen in the lacrimal gland when compared to the orbit.
2. Symptoms and Signs: The patient presents usually with painless mass in the lacrimal gland region. On palpation, the tumor is firm in consistency with typical S-shaped configuration [28–30].
3. Differential Diagnoses: Benign and malignant lacrimal gland tumors.

Eyelid OAL

1. Eyelid OAL comprises 5% of OALs and is located in the preseptal region. It is commonly seen in elderly population with slight male preponderance.

2. Clinical Presentation: It is commonly seen in the upper eyelid and is characterized by soft rubbery mass. Levator muscle infiltration is seen in 10% of the cases. Most of these lymphomas are of B-cell type [31–36].
3. Differential Diagnoses: Granulomatous diseases, neural tumors, vascular tumors, and xanthogranuloma.

Lacrimal sac OAL

1. Lacrimal sac OAL comprises <5% of OALs. In contrast to orbital OALs, the incidence of EMZL and DLBCL is equally common.
2. Clinical Presentation: Patients with lacrimal sac OAL usually present with lacrimal sac swelling, watering, chronic dacryocystitis, or sometimes blood-stained tears [37, 38].
3. Differential Diagnosis: Primary acquired naso-lacrimal duct obstruction.

Association with Intraocular Lymphoma

Intraocular uveal lymphoma has the tendency to spread through the perivascular and perineural areas transsclerally and is associated with ocular adnexal extension in <35% of cases [39].

Systemic Association

Though multiple predictors of systemic lymphoma like pathologic criteria, immunophenotype, and genetic analysis have been described, laterality and anatomical location of the lymphoma are found to be more helpful in predicting the development of systemic spread. The risk is more for bilateral OALs (72% in orbital, 47% in conjunctival OAL) when compared to the unilateral ones (12% in orbital, 17% in conjunctival OAL). Eyelid OAL (70%) is a significant predictor of systemic lymphoma followed by orbital (35%) and conjunctival OAL (20%). Systemic evaluation is recommended for all the patients with OAL twice yearly as the risk increases from <10% at 1 year to >30% at 10 years. The most frequently involved sites are lymph nodes followed by gut (19%), bone marrow (8%), brain (6%), lung (3%). The associated symptoms are fever, malaise, fatigue, weight loss, termed as B symptoms historically, though the term is obsolete now [40, 41].

Imaging

1. Anterior Segment OCT (AS-OCT): AS-OCT is helpful for bulbar conjunctival lymphomas of <4 mm thickness. Conjunctival OAL is characterized by sub-epithelial hyporeflective lesion with densely arranged hyperreflective stroma on AS-OCT [42].
2. Computed Tomography (CT Scan):

   Indications:

   It is used as primary modality in the diagnosis of ocular adnexal lymphomas. It helps in localizing the tumor in orbit and also assists in surgical planning. Imaging helps in identifying the orbital extension of the tumor in conjunctiva and eyelid OALs with subclinical orbital disease.

   Location: The most common location noted on imaging is orbit (78%) followed by conjunctiva (9%), lacrimal sac (9%), and eyelid (5%).

   Typical Features: Lymphomas appear as localized masses with well-defined margins. The tumor is well circumscribed, homogeneous, and hyperdense to isodense. It is characterized by the lesion molding the globe and the soft tissue structures in the orbit because of its cellular composition. This arrangement is called "casting sign" or "ring sign." As the tumor spreads along the fascial planes like a pancake pattern, it is also described as an oblong tumor. With the administration of contrast agent, the tumor is homogeneous with intake of moderate to marked amount of contrast.

   The region of the distribution includes preseptal region in eyelid OAL, confined to lacrimal gland or involving the retrobulbar region which can be localized to one or more quadrants or diffuse in orbital type without any bony involvement [43].

   Atypical Features: High-grade lymphomas like DLBCL, mantle cell lymphomas are rapidly progressive and infiltrate the orbital soft tissues causing globe indentation, appear heterogeneous, with infiltration of adjacent bony structures. Bony changes include irregular bony margins and erosions. CT is the preferred imaging modality for orbital lymphomas as the bony changes are well delineated when compared to magnetic resonance imaging (MRI) [44].

3. Magnetic Resonance Imaging (MRI): MRI imaging modality is usually confined to the tumors with local spread to the paranasal sinuses, or with intracranial extension or with optic nerve infiltration causing diagnostic dilemma. The tumor is isointense on T1 and T2 weighted images. With gadolinium contrast, the tumor shows moderate enhancement on MRI [19, 44].

Conclusion

Lymphomas are the most common malignant tumors in ocular adnexa. They most commonly involve the orbit followed by conjunctiva and rarely involve the eyelid. Adnexal lymphomas are predominantly EMZL type of B-cell lymphomas with good prognosis. AS-OCT is helpful in differentiating conjunctival lymphomas from the simulating conjunctival lesions. CT orbits are the preferred imaging modality to define the tumor extent and bony changes if any. MRI orbits are useful in adnexal lymphomas extending beyond the orbit or those involving the optic nerve (Figs. 5.1, 5.2, and 5.3).

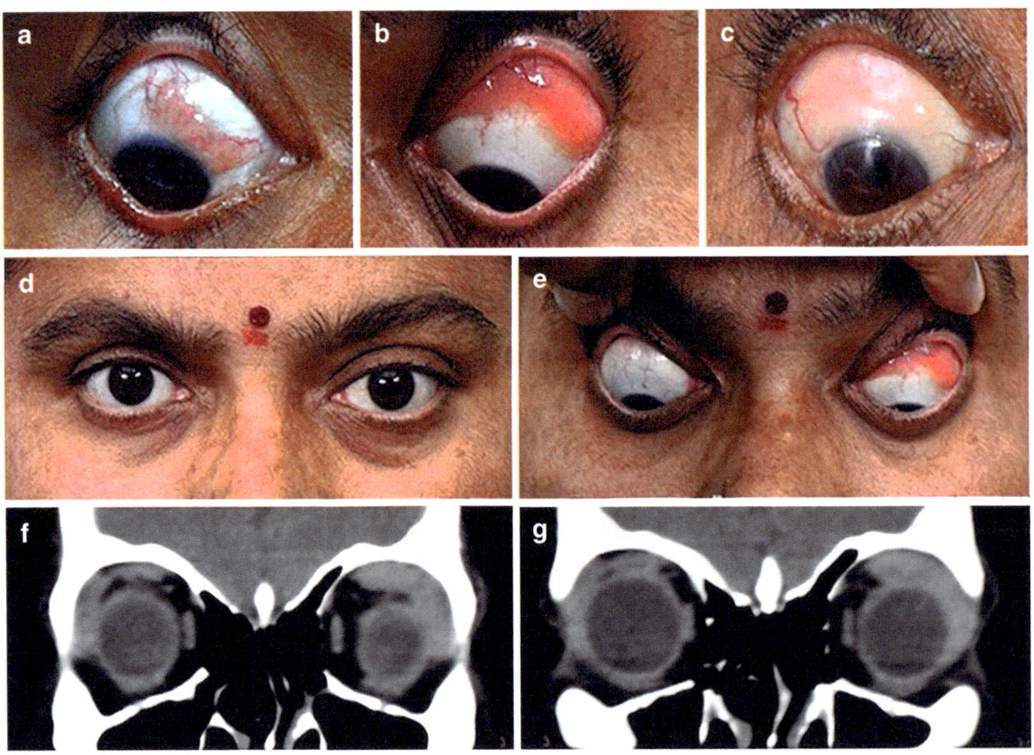

Fig. 5.1 Conjunctival lymphoma. Conjunctival lymphoma is characterized by "Salmon color patch," a subconjunctival pink fleshy mass and presents as (**a**) bulbar or (**b**) forniceal or (**c**) diffusely located subconjunctival mass. (**d**) Clinical photograph of middle-aged female patient with left eye ptosis. (**e**) On upper eyelid elevation, pinkish forniceal mass was identified with (**f**, **g**) orbital extension on imaging

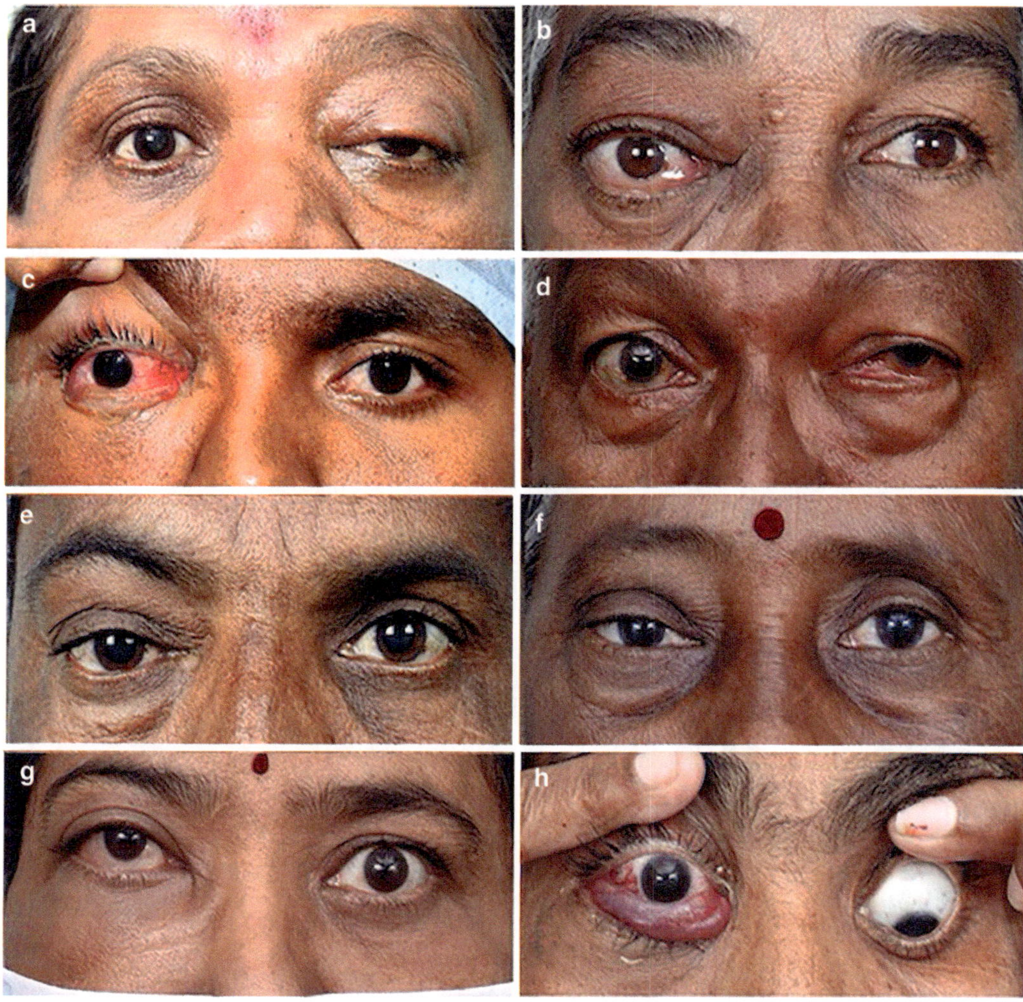

Fig. 5.2 Varied presentation of ocular adnexal lymphoma. Clinical photographs showing the wide variety of clinical presentation including (**a**) left eye ptosis, (**b**) right eye proptosis, (**c**) redness in right eye, (**d**) palpable mass in left lower eyelid of left eye, (**e**) fullness in superior sulcus of right eye, (**f**) periorbital swelling of right eye, (**g**) upward displacement of right eye, (**h**) limited movement of right eye in down gaze

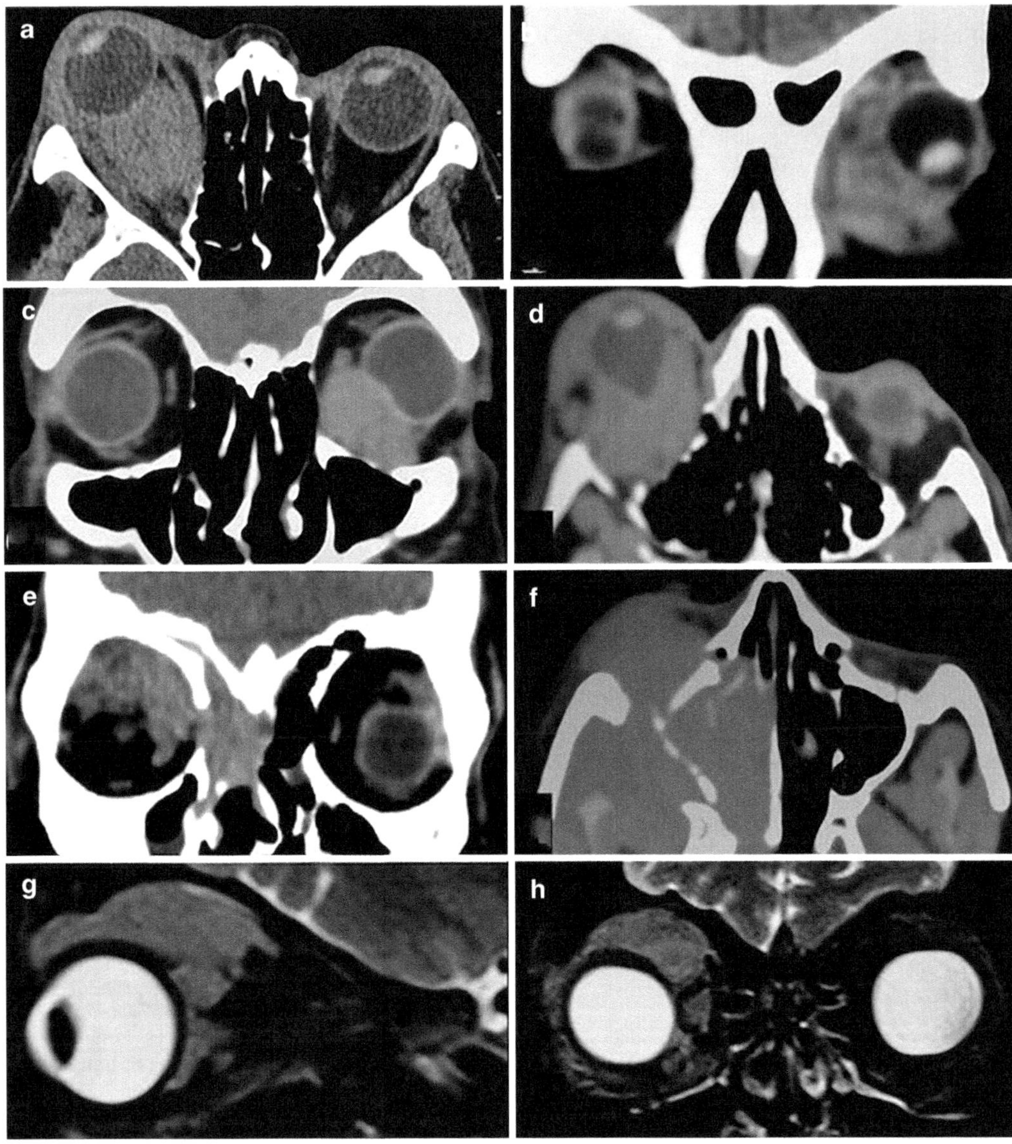

Fig. 5.3 Orbital imaging features of ocular adnexal lymphoma. (**a**) Computed tomography of the orbit axial sections showing well-defined isodense lesion molding around the right globe in the intraconal space. (**b**) Similar arrangement of the lesion is seen in coronal cuts of the left eye called "casting sign" or "ring sign." (**c**, **d**) Atypical presentation of high-grade lymphomas with globe indentation and with (**e**, **f**) infiltration of adjacent bone. (**g**) Sagittal and (**h**) coronal sections of magnetic resonance T2 weighted images of the right orbit showing isointense lesion molding around the globe predominantly in the extraconal space of the superior orbit with minimal intraconal component of the lesion

References

1. Bardenstein DS. Orbital and adnexal lymphoma. In: Singh A, et al., editors. Clinical ophthalmic oncology. Philadelphia, PA: Saunders-Elsevier; 2007. p. 565–70.
2. Sjo LD. Ophthalmic lymphoma: epidemiology and pathogenesis. Acta Ophthalmol. 2009;87(1):1–20.
3. Sjo LD, Ralfkiaer E, Prause JU, et al. Increasing incidence of ophthalmic lymphoma in Denmark from 1980 to 2005. Invest Ophthalmol Vis Sci. 2008;49(8):3283–8.
4. Carbone PP, Kaplan HS, Musshoff K, et al. Report of the Committee on Hodgkin's disease staging classification. Cancer Res. 1971;31:1860–1.
5. Heegaard S, Chevez-Barrios P, White VA, Coupland SE, Finger PT. Ocular Adnexal lymphoma. In: Amin MB, Edge SB, Greene FL, Byrd DR, Brookland RK, Washington MK, et al., editors. AJCC cancer staging manual. 8th ed. Cham: Springer International Publishing; 2017. p. 849–54.
6. Coupland SE, White VA, Rootman JE, et al. A TNM-based clinical staging system of ocular adnexal lymphomas. Arch Pathol Lab Med. 2009;133:1262–7.
7. Cheson BD, Fisher RI, Barrington SF, et al. Recommendations for initial evaluation, staging, and response assessment of Hodgkin and non-Hodgkin lymphoma: the Lugano classification. J Clin Oncol. 2014;32(27):3059–68.
8. Cheson BD, Ansell S, Schwartz L, et al. Refinement of the Lugano Classification lymphoma response criteria in the era of immunomodulatory therapy. Blood. 2016;128(21):2489–96.
9. Sjö LD. Ophthalmic lymphoma: epidemiology and pathogenesis. Acta Ophthalmol. 2009;87(1):1–20.
10. Li JJ, Chen W, Sadeghi N. Conjunctival lymphoma. BMJ Case Rep. 2019;12(7):e229599.
11. Calvo R, Ribera JM, Vaquero M, et al. Low-grade, malt-type, primary B-cell lymphoma of the conjunctiva. Leuk Lymphoma. 1997;28(1–2):203–7.
12. Rubin PAD, Kent CJ, Jakobiec FA. Orbital and ocular adnexal lymphoid tumors: Albert & Jakobiec's principles and practice of ophthalmology. 3rd ed. St Louis, MO: WB Saunders Company, Elsevier; 2018.
13. Ferry JA, Fung CY, Zukerberg L, et al. Lymphoma of the ocular adnexa: a study of 353 cases. Am J Surg Pathol. 2007;31(2):170–84.
14. Oh DE, Kim YD. Lymphoproliferative diseases of the ocular adnexa in Korea. Arch Ophthalmol. 2007;125(12):1668–73.
15. Ozkan MC, Palamar M, Tombuloglu M, et al. Ocular adnexal lymphomas: single-center experience. Clin Lymphoma Myeloma Leuk. 2015;15(Suppl):S158–60.
16. Streubel B, Lamprecht A, Dierlamm J, et al. T(14;18)(q32;q21) involving IGH and MALT1 is a frequent chromosomal aberration in MALT lymphoma. Blood. 2003;101:2335–9.
17. Streubel B, Vinatzer U, Lamprecht A, Raderer M, Chott A. T(3; 14)(p14.1;q32) involving IGH and FOXP1 is a novel recurrent chromosomal aberration in MALT lymphoma. Leukemia. 2005;19:652–8.
18. Verdijk RM. Lymphoproliferative tumors of the ocular adnexa. Asia Pac J Ophthalmol. 2017;6(2):132–42.
19. Shields JA, Saunders WB. Lymphoid tumors and leukemias. Diagnosis and management of orbital tumors. 1st ed. Philadelphia, PA: J.B. Lippincott; 1989.
20. Watkins LM, Carter KD, Nerad JA. Ocular adnexal lymphoma of the extraocular muscles: case series from the University of Iowa and review of the literature. Ophthal Plast Reconstr Surg. 2011;27:471–6.
21. Gill MK, Jampol LM. Variations in the presentation of primary intraocular lymphoma: case reports and a review. Surv Ophthalmol. 2001;45:463–71.
22. Kuro M, Matsuyama K, Matsuoka M, et al. Case of primary intraocular lymphoma with extraocular extension. Ocul Oncol Pathol. 2015;2(2):66–70.
23. Demirci H, Shields C, Shields J, et al. Orbital tumors in the older adult population. Ophthalmology. 2002;109:243–8.
24. Coupland SE, Damato B. Lymphomas involving the eye and the ocular adnexa. Curr Opin Ophthalmol. 2006;17:523–31.
25. Knowles DM, Jakobiec FA, McNally L, et al. Lymphoid hyperplasia and malignant lymphoma occurring in the ocular adnexa (orbit, conjunctiva, and eyelids): a prospective multiparametric analysis of 108 cases during 1977 to 1987. Hum Pathol. 1990;21:959–73.
26. Olsen TG, Heegaard S. Orbital lymphoma. Surv Ophthalmol. 2019;64(1):45–66.
27. Charton J, Witherspoon SR, Itani K, et al. Natural killer/T-cell lymphoma masquerading as orbital cellulitis. Ophthal Plast Reconstr Surg. 2008;24(2):143–5.
28. Cassidy DT, McKelvie P, Harris GJ, et al. Lacrimal gland orbital lobe cysts associated with MALT lymphoma and primary Sjogren's syndrome. Orbit. 2005;24(4):257–63.
29. Coupland SE, Foss HD, Hummel M, et al. Extranodal marginal zone B-cell lymphoma of the lacrimal gland associated with crystal-storing histiocytosis. Ophthalmology. 2002;109(1):105–10.
30. Bertelmann E, Minko N. Safety of the preoperative evaluation of pleomorphic adenoma: a retrospective analysis. Klin Monatsbl Augenheilkd. 2012;229(3):231–5.
31. Coupland SE, Hellmich M, Auw-Haedrich C, et al. Prognostic value of cell-cycle markers in ocular adnexal lymphoma: an assessment of 230 cases. Graefes Arch Clin Exp Ophthalmol. 2004;242:130–45.
32. Coupland SE, Krause L, Delecluse HJ, et al. Lymphoproliferative lesions of the ocular adnexa. Analysis of 112 cases. Ophthalmology. 1998;105:1430–41.

33. Fung CY, Tarbell NJ, Lucarelli MJ, et al. Ocular adnexal lymphoma: clinical behavior of distinct World Health Organization classification subtypes. Int J Radiat Oncol Biol Phys. 2003;57:1382–91.
34. McKelvie PA, McNab A, Francis IC, et al. Ocular adnexal lymphoproliferative disease: a series of 73 cases. Clin Exp Ophthalmol. 2001;29:387–93.
35. Meunier J, Lumbroso-Le Rouic L, Vincent-Salomon A, et al. Ophthalmologic and intraocular non-Hodgkin's lymphoma: a large single centre study of initial characteristics, natural history, and prognostic factors. Hematol Oncol. 2004;22:143–58.
36. Sullivan TJ, Whitehead K, Williamson R, et al. Lymphoproliferative disease of the ocular adnexa: a clinical and pathologic study with statistical analysis of 69 patients. Ophthal Plast Reconstr Surg. 2005;21:177–88.
37. Alkatan HM, Alaraj A, El-Khani A, et al. Ocular adnexal lymphoproliferative disorders in an ophthalmic referral center in Saudi Arabia. Saudi J Ophthalmol. 2013;27:227–30.
38. Berry-Brincat A, Tomlins P, Hall A, et al. Primary extrasac orbital lymphoma presenting as nasolacrimal obstruction. Orbit. 2008;27(3):175–7.
39. Mashayekhi A, Shukla SY, Shields JA, et al. Choroidal lymphoma: clinical features and association with systemic lymphoma. Ophthalmology. 2014;121(1):342–51.
40. Shields CL, Shields JA, Carvalho C, Rundle P, Smith AF. Conjunctival lymphoid tumors: clinical analysis of 117 cases and relationship to systemic lymphoma. Ophthalmology. 2001;108(5):979–84.
41. Demirci H, Shields CL, Karatza EC, et al. Orbital lymphoproliferative tumors: analysis of clinical features and systemic involvement in 160 cases. Ophthalmology. 2008;115(9):1626–31.
42. Vempuluru VS, Jakati S, Godbole A, et al. Spectrum of AS-OCT features of ocular surface tumors and correlation of clinico-tomographic features with histopathology: a study of 70 lesions. Int Ophthalmol. 2021;41(11):3571–86.
43. Naik MN, Tourani KL, Sekhar GC, et al. Interpretation of computed tomography imaging of the eye and orbit: a systematic approach. Indian J Ophthalmol. 2002;50:339–53.
44. Sullivan TJ, Valenzuela AA. Imaging features of ocular adnexal lymphoproliferative disease. Eye. 2006;20:1189–95.

Intraocular Lymphoma: Clinical Presentation and Imaging Studies

6

Kedarisetti Kiran Chandra and Vishal R. Raval

Primary Vitreoretinal Lymphoma/PCNSL-O

Introduction

Primary central nervous system lymphoma (PCNSL) is a subtype of non-Hodgkin lymphoma confined to the CNS compartments. As per the 2017 World Health Organization classification of hematopoietic and lymphoid tumors, PCNSL is classified as primary diffuse large B-cell lymphoma (DLBCL) of the CNS [1]. The CNS compartments include the brain (deep cortical regions, periventricular regions, and basal ganglia), spinal cord, meninges, and the eyes [2]. Primary intraocular lymphoma is a malignant neoplasm derived from monoclonal proliferations of B- or T-lymphocytes and is classified according to its location into either primary vitreoretinal lymphoma or primary uveal lymphoma. PCNSL-O is the preferred term for vitreoretinal lymphoma to emphasize that it is an ocular variant or subset of primary CNS lymphoma (PCNSL). Those with concurrent CNS and ocular disease may be labeled as (PCNSL-CNS/O) in contrast to patients with CNS only involvement (PCNSL-CNS) at presentation. The involvement of the eye and other CNS compartments varies as ophthalmic manifestations can precede, occur simultaneously with or follow disease in other CNS sites. Sixty percent to 90% of patients with PCNSL-O ultimately involve other CNS compartments, while 20% of patients with PCNSL present with concurrent PCNSL-O [3, 4]. The PCNSL-O often masquerades as infection or inflammation leading to a delay in diagnosis and inappropriate management.

K. K. Chandra
Anant Bajaj Retina Institute, L V Prasad Eye Institute, Hyderabad, Telangana, India

V. R. Raval (✉)
Anant Bajaj Retina Institute, The Operation Eyesight Universal Institute for Eye Cancer, L V Prasad Eye Institute, Hyderabad, Telangana, India

Epidemiology

Most patients of PCNSL-O are older than 40 years with the usual age of onset being in the late 50s and 60s [5]. The Central Brain Tumor Registry of the U.S. noted an incidence of PCNSL to peak between 75 and 84 years. Most reports of PCNSL-O have found increased incidence in females than in males, in contrast to PCNSL which tends to occur in higher frequency in males [6, 7]. PCNSL-O may be either unilateral or bilateral on initial presentation, but approximately 80–90% of patients will ultimately develop bilateral disease [8, 9]. The median interval between the progression of lymphoma from the eye to other CNS compartments and vice versa varies over a follow-up of 8–29 months [3, 9–11]. In a recent review by Farrall et al. the

V. R. Raval et al. (eds.), *Ocular and Adnexal Lymphoma*, Essentials in Ophthalmology,
https://doi.org/10.1007/978-3-031-24595-4_6

prevalence of ocular involvement at any time during the course of PCNSL was 16% with greater prevalence (69%) of CNS involvement with ocular involvement [2].

Clinical Presentation

Majority of patients often complain of painless loss of vision and floaters. The rest of the patients are asymptomatic or diagnosed during ophthalmic screening in the setting of known PCNSL. Few rare presentations include exudative retinal detachment, elevated posterior pole lesion, neovascularization, optic neuropathy, and a variety of chorioretinal abnormalities [12].

Ophthalmic examination of anterior segment is usually unremarkable; however, few patients may present with corneal precipitates or mild anterior flare. Chronic waxing and waning course of uveitis may simulate pseudo-hypopyon formation, neovascularization of iris, and secondary glaucoma. Secondary infiltration of the anterior segment may lead to mass formation in the angle or iris. PCNSL-O with T cell variant presents with severe anterior segment inflammation and keratic precipitates [13].

Posterior segment typically presents with significant vitreous inflammation and vitreous cells. The cells typically associated with PCNSL-O are larger than inflammatory cells and organize into strands, clumps, or sheets along with the vitreous fibrils. The lymphoma cells lining along the vitreous gives characteristic "aurora borealis" like appearance [3, 14]. Fundus examination exhibits hallmark features of a flat creamy orange–yellow lesion seen deeper within the sensory retina (Fig. 6.1a, c). Lesions may be single or multiple, confluent or discrete, and may appear as multiple punctate lesions [8, 9, 12]. The presence of multiple subretinal punctate lesions secondary to sub-RPE infiltration with lymphoma cells also known as "leopard spots" is a common finding seen in majority of cases [3] (Fig. 6.2a). Rarely the patient may present with retinal hemorrhages or a single solitary intraocular mass [15]. Associated features include retinal vasculitis, exudative retinal detachment, retinal pigment epithelial atrophy with subretinal fibrosis, disciform scarring, and optic nerve infiltration.

CNS lesions may lead to focal or general symptoms. Generalized signs of increased intracranial pressure (ICP) or more focal symptoms such as weakness, sensory deficits, or aphasia should be evaluated [16].

Diagnosis

Although clinical examination and ocular imaging are of help in the diagnosis of PCNSL-O, the histopathology examination of the ocular specimens, with demonstration of malignant B lymphocytes in the vitreous or retina still remains the gold standard test to confirm the diagnosis. Immunohistochemistry to characterize lymphocyte type and clonality aids in the management.

Optical Coherence Tomography (OCT)

The lymphoma cells directly infiltrate the retina and proliferate focally in the pre-Bruch's/sub-RPE space corresponding to the lesions seen on clinical examination as subretinal precipitates.

The typical presenting feature of lymphoma on OCT is the presence of nodular or band hyperreflective spots noted in the pre-Bruch's or sub-RPE space [17, 18] (Fig. 6.1d, e). The infiltrations can be subtle RPE hyperreflective mottling, focal discrete hyperreflective nodularity under RPE or retina, large hyperreflective lesions that create confluent bands of material under the retina, or solid RPE detachments [17, 19].

SD-OCT features such as RPE damage, disruption of the photoreceptor inner segment/outer segment junction, multiple hyperreflective infiltrations in the inner retina, and exudative retinal detachment with subretinal hyporeflective fluid are described in cases with severe PCNSL-O [20]. Vertical hyperreflective lesions extending from the outer to the inner retina have also been described which often preceded the development of subretinal pigment epithelial deposits. In most cases, they resolved with minimal or no scarring after the initiation of chemotherapy [17, 21].

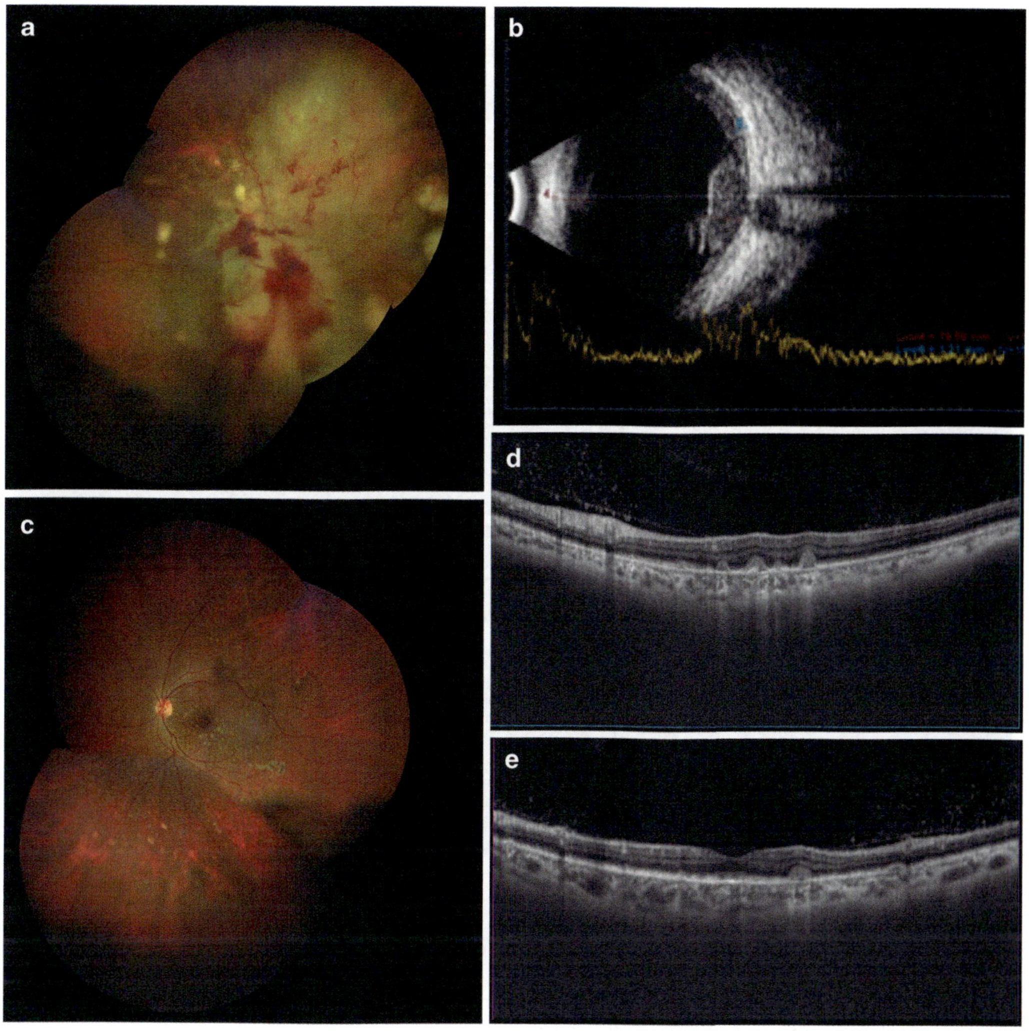

Fig. 6.1 A 55-year-old woman complaining of diminution of vision associated with floaters in the right eye. Fundus photograph of right eye shows a creamy yellowish elevated lesion at the posterior involving the optic disc with retinal hemorrhages (**a**). The corresponding B-scan demonstrated an elevated subretinal lesion involving the optic nerve head with diffuse flat hyperechoic lesions infiltrating the subretinal space and significant dot echoes in the vitreous cavity (**b**). Fundus photograph of the left eye shows multiple creamy white deposits involving the retinal layers (**c**). Optical coherence tomography shows multiple hyperreflective dots in the vitreous cavity along with nodular hyperreflective elevated lesions underneath the retinal pigment epithelium (RPE) (**d**, **e**)

A study by Dalvin et al. has reported 43% of PCNSL-O eyes have sub-RPE deposits and proposed to be a marker of recurrence, poor visual prognosis, and lower survival time [19]. However, a clear association has not been established. The sub-RPE deposits resolve with chemotherapy and hence OCT is a valuable tool to monitor treatment and to observe for relapse/resolution of PCNSL-O [22].

Fundus Autofluorescence (FAF)

Fundus autofluorescence demonstrates hypo-autofluorescence corresponding to areas of RPE atrophy and hyper-autofluorescence corresponding to areas with lymphoma cell infiltration [18, 23] (Fig. 6.2b). On multimodal imaging, hyper autofluorescent spots seen on FAF may correlate with the hypofluorescent spots seen on fluorescein angiography (FA; 36%) and the nodular

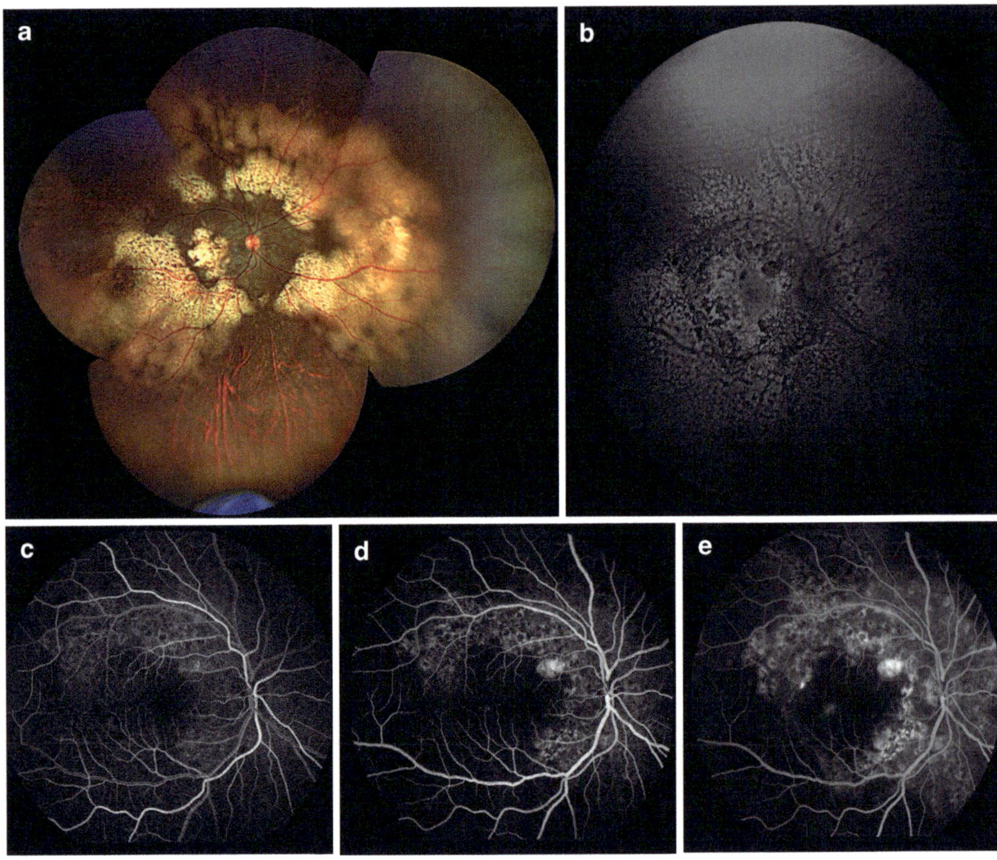

Fig. 6.2 A 60-year-old man complained of diminution of vision in the right eye. Fundus photograph of the right eye shows ill-defined creamy lesions with yellowish infiltrates located deep in the retina giving a characteristic "leopard skin" pigmentation overlying the lesion (**a**). Fundus autofluorescence shows areas of hypo- with hyper-autofluorescence in the posterior pole (**b**). Fluorescein angiography in early, mid, and late phase shows numerous small hypofluorescent lesions corresponding to punctate yellowish lesions in the fundus with few areas of staining in the late phase corresponding to RPE atrophy (**c**–**e**)

hyperreflective spots on OCT (43%) [24]. This concordance was observed in 62% of patients. FAF can also be a valuable tool to document the progression of the disease as well as prognosticate the patient considering the hyper-autofluorescence lesions become hypo following complete resolution of the lesions [25].

B-scan Ultrasound (USG)

B-scan USG is useful to document clusters of condensed punctate echoes as well as elevated chorioretinal lesions and optic nerve widening [26, 27] (Fig. 6.1b).

Fundus Fluorescein Angiography (FA)

On FA, hypofluorescent spots may represent retinal lymphomatous infiltrates, whereas hyperfluorescent spots represent atrophic lesions secondary to RPE window defects [18] (Fig. 6.2c–e). The punctate hyperfluorescent window defects and hypofluorescent lesions give a characteristic "leopard spot" appearance. In late phase of the disease staining at the level of the RPE may be seen [28].

Indocyanine Green Angiography (ICGA)

ICGA often shows round clustered hypocyanescent lesions corresponding to the areas of hypofluorescence seen on FA, but it may be completely normal or non-contributory [18, 29]. Other associated features such as perivascular staining or leakage, cystoid macular edema or optic nerve head staining or leakage, are unusual in PCNSL-O and help to distinguish it from patients with chronic uveitis or vitritis of non-malignant etiology.

Disease Staging

Staging evaluation for the patient is an important part of management. It is usually done in patients with biopsy confirmed diagnosis of PCNSL-O to rule out extraocular sites of involvement like the CNS or testis. MRI brain with contrast along with lumbar puncture for cerebrospinal fluid (CSF) evaluation should be obtained in all patients diagnosed with PCNSL-O since 80% of these patients ultimately develop lymphoma in other areas of their central nervous system [30]. Neurological lesions appear hypo-dense on T1-weighted, hyper-dense on T2-weighted scans with discrete or diffuse borders with characteristic dense and diffuse contrast enhancement. Meningeal enhancement with gadolinium contrast is indicative of leptomeningeal dissemination (LMD). Testicular ultrasound can also be considered in male patients, as the testes represent a relatively immune privileged site where lymphoma can be detected [31]. Serological testing for HIV, hepatitis B and C, plus quantification of serum lactate dehydrogenase (LDH) should also be considered as standard-of-care at baseline.

Diagnostic Biopsy

Biopsy for the cytological assessment of suspected PCNSL-O is invaluable not only in confirming the diagnosis but also in providing information of prognostic importance [32, 33]. The biopsy specimen can be obtained either from vitreous or subretinal infiltrates and processed for cytological, immunological, and genetic studies [34, 35]. This will be described in detail in the chapter on intraocular biopsy techniques.

Differential Diagnosis

PCNSL-O is a great masquerader and hence should be distinguished from other infectious and non-infectious uveitic entities such as tuberculosis, sarcoidosis, viral retinitis, retinochoroidal toxoplasmosis, syphilitic retinitis, endophthalmitis, or idiopathic uveitis that present with vitreous cells. The sub-RPE deposits seen on OCT should be differentiated from those seen in age related macular degeneration, polypoidal vasculopathy, and chronic central serous chorioretinopathy. Other neoplastic etiologies such as choroidal metastasis and amelanotic choroidal melanoma can also rarely simulate PCNSL-O lesions.

Primary Uveal Lymphoma

Introduction

Unlike PCNSL-O, primary uveal lymphoma is often unilateral and has a benign, indolent course. It is typically a non-Hodgkin's lymphoma, most frequently of B-cell origin. The predominant subtype is extra-nodal marginal zone B-cell lymphoma (EMZL) or mucosa-associated lymphoid tissue (MALT) [36, 37].

Clinical Features

Patients complain of painless diminution of vision or metamorphopsia due to retinal detachment. They may present with raised intraocular pressure or proptosis when extraocular involvement occurs. Salmon color patches may be seen if subconjunctival or episcleral involvement occurs. Fundus examination shows multifocal yellow-white choroidal infiltration in the early stages and diffuse choroidal thickening in the later stages of the disease [37] (Fig. 6.3a). Choroidal folds and placoid infiltrates may also be seen. The fundus location of these findings is

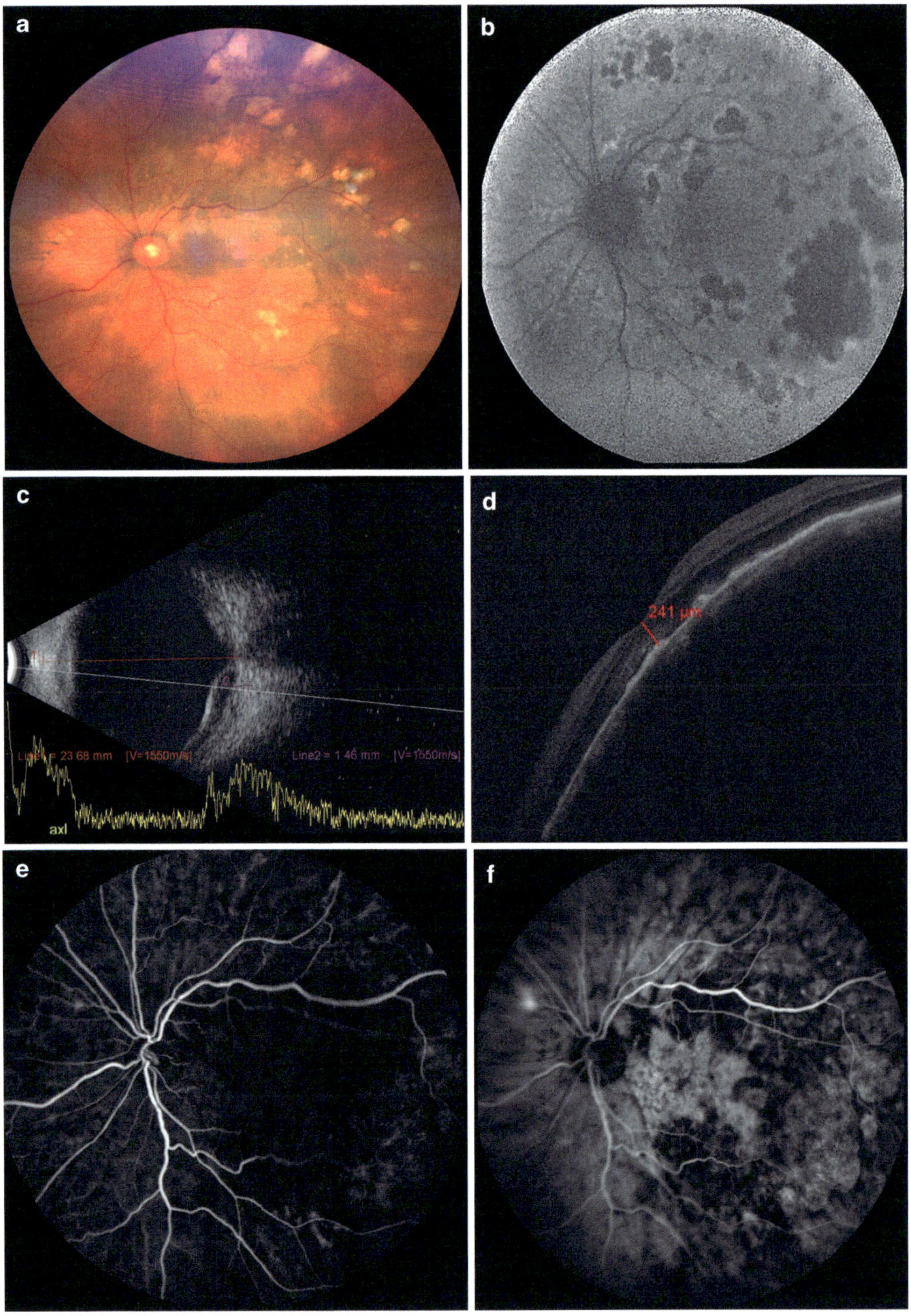

Fig. 6.3 A 52-year-old woman complained of sudden diminution of vision in the left eye. Fundus photograph of the left eye shows multifocal, yellow choroidal infiltrates involving the posterior pole associated with choroidal thickening (**a**). Fundus autofluorescence shows multiple areas of hypo- with hyper-autofluorescence lesions (**b**). B-scan ultrasound shows diffuse choroidal thickening without extrascleral extension (**c**). Optical coherence tomography shows an elevated choroidal lesion with minimal subretinal fluid and photoreceptor loss (**d**). Indocyanine green angiography in the early and late phase demonstrated hypocyanescent areas corresponding to areas of choroidal infiltrates and hypercyanescent areas in the late phase corresponding to RPE atrophy (**e**, **f**)

typically anterior to the arcades [37]. Vitreous is often clear at presentation. CNS involvement is rare and seen only in advanced disease stages.

Diagnosis

Diagnosis is usually challenging considering the rare presentation of the disease. Ultrasonography imaging shows a discrete mass with relatively smooth-surface, diffuse choroidal thickening, or presence of subretinal fluid [37] (Fig. 6.3c). B-scan ultrasound is also helpful to detect frank extrascleral extension.

SD-OCT features of choroidal lymphoma show lumpy bumpy choroid with varying topography and increased tumor thickness [38]. Arias et al. have described marked thickening of the choroid with striking choroidal surface undulation and folds imparting an appearance similar to a "sea storm" (seasick appearance) [39] (Fig. 6.3d). Mild tumor infiltration of choroid shows uniform choroidal surface, medium infiltration appears rippled, and thick infiltration appears undulated [40].

Fundus autofluorescence shows multiple areas of hypo- with hyper-autofluorescence lesions corresponding to areas of active choroidal infiltrations and overlying RPE atrophy (Fig. 6.3b). Fluorescein angiography demonstrates early hyperfluorescence in most cases. Few patients have choroidal folds and hypofluorescent spots corresponding to the clinically observed choroidal infiltrates on FA. Indocyanine green angiography reveals hypofluorescent lesions corresponding to the clinically observed choroidal infiltrates [37] (Fig. 6.3e, f).

Differential Diagnosis

The diagnosis of PUL is challenging as it can simulate other benign and malignant conditions such as choroidal hemangioma, posterior scleritis, uveal effusion syndrome, sarcoidosis, choroidal metastasis, and amelanotic choroidal melanoma. Multimodal imaging and biopsy help to confirm the diagnosis.

Conclusion

PCNSL-O diagnosis remains challenging, with vague signs and symptoms and difficult diagnostic confirmation. Appropriate suspicion of chronic, treatment-resistant uveitis can aid in earlier detection. Definitive diagnosis still requires the identification of lymphoma cells from the vitreous or subretinal space in case of PCNSL-O and choroid or extraorbital sites in case of uveal lymphoma. Systemic screening and neuroimaging at presentation and follow-up is mandatory considering concurrent or subsequent CNS involvement seen in patients with PCNSL-O.

Financial Disclosure None.

Conflict of Interest None.

Funding Source This work was supported by The Operation Eyesight Universal Institute for Eye Cancer and Hyderabad Eye Research Foundation, Hyderabad, India.

References

1. Grimm SA, Pulido JS, Jahnke K, Schiff D, Hall AJ, Shenkier TN, et al. Primary intraocular lymphoma: an International Primary Central Nervous System Lymphoma Collaborative Group Report. Ann Oncol. 2007;18(11):1851–5.
2. Farrall AL, Smith JR. Eye involvement in primary central nervous system lymphoma. Surv Ophthalmol. 2020;65:548.
3. Chan CC, Rubenstein JL, Coupland SE, Davis JL, Harbour JW, Johnston PB, et al. Primary vitreoretinal lymphoma: a report from an International Primary Central Nervous System Lymphoma Collaborative Group symposium. Oncologist. 2011;16(11):1589–99.
4. Hochberg FH, Miller DC. Primary central nervous system lymphoma. J Neurosurg. 1988;68(6):835–53.
5. Mochizuki M, Singh AD. Epidemiology and clinical features of intraocular lymphoma. Ocul Immunol Inflamm. 2009;17(2):69–72.
6. Coupland SE, Damato B. Understanding intraocular lymphomas. Clin Exp Ophthalmol. 2008;36(6):564–78.
7. Sen HN, Bodaghi B, Hoang PL, Nussenblatt R. Primary intraocular lymphoma: diagnosis and differential diagnosis. Ocul Immunol Inflamm. 2009;17(3):133–41.
8. Coupland SE, Heimann H, Bechrakis NE. Primary intraocular lymphoma: a review of the clini-

cal, histopathological and molecular biological features. Graefes Arch Clin Exp Ophthalmol. 2004;242(11):901–13.
9. Char DH, Ljung BM, Miller T, Phillips T. Primary intraocular lymphoma (ocular reticulum cell sarcoma) diagnosis and management. Ophthalmology. 1988;95(5):625–30.
10. Sagoo MS, Mehta H, Swampillai AJ, Cohen VM, Amin SZ, Plowman PN, et al. Primary intraocular lymphoma. Surv Ophthalmol. 2014;59(5):503–16.
11. Raval V, Binkley E, Aronow ME, Valenzuela J, Peereboom DM, Singh AD. Primary central nervous system lymphoma - ocular variant: an interdisciplinary review on management. Surv Ophthalmol. 2021;66(6):1009–20.
12. Freeman LN, Schachat AP, Knox DL, Michels RG, Green WR. Clinical features, laboratory investigations, and survival in ocular reticulum cell sarcoma. Ophthalmology. 1987;94(12):1631–9.
13. Abu Samra K, Oray M, Ebrahimiadib N, Lee S, Anesi S, Foster CS. Intraocular lymphoma: descriptive data of 26 patients including clinico-pathologic features, vitreous findings, and treatment outcomes. Ocul Immunol Inflamm. 2018;26(3):347–52.
14. Chan CC, Wallace DJ. Intraocular lymphoma: update on diagnosis and management. Cancer Control. 2004;11(5):285–95.
15. Fredrick DR, Char DH, Ljung BM, Brinton DA. Solitary intraocular lymphoma as an initial presentation of widespread disease. Arch Ophthalmol. 1989;107(3):395–7.
16. Doucet S, Kumthekar P, Raizer J. Primary central nervous system lymphoma. Curr Treat Options in Oncol. 2013;14(2):185–97.
17. Barry RJ, Tasiopoulou A, Murray PI, Patel PJ, Sagoo MS, Denniston AK. Characteristic optical coherence tomography findings in patients with primary vitreoretinal lymphoma: a novel aid to early diagnosis. Br J Ophthalmol. 2018;102(10):1362–6.
18. Lavine JA, Singh AD, Sharma S, Baynes K, Lowder CY, Srivastava SK. Ultra-widefield multimodal imaging of primary vitreoretinal lymphoma. Retina. 2019;39(10):1861–71.
19. Dalvin LA, Lim LS, Ancona-Lezama D, Mazloumi M, Chang M, Mashayekhi A, et al. Tumor control and visual acuity outcomes in vitreoretinal lymphoma with and without sub-retinal pigment epithelium infiltration: analysis of 125 eyes of 70 patients at a single ocular oncology center. Ophthalmol Retina. 2019;3(11):998–1005.
20. Yang X, Dalvin LA, Mazloumi M, Ferenczy S, Lim LS, Ancona-Lezama D, et al. Spectral domain optical coherence tomography features of vitreoretinal lymphoma in 55 eyes. Retina. 2021;41(2):249–58.
21. Deák GG, Goldstein DA, Zhou M, Fawzi AA, Jampol LM. Vertical hyperreflective lesions on optical coherence tomography in vitreoretinal lymphoma. JAMA Ophthalmol. 2019;137(2):194–8.
22. Zhao H, Wang X, Mao Y, Peng X. Longitudinal observation of OCT imaging is a valuable tool to monitor primary vitreoretinal lymphoma treated with intravitreal injections of methotrexate. BMC Ophthalmol. 2020;20(1):10.
23. Casady M, Faia L, Nazemzadeh M, Nussenblatt R, Chan CC, Sen HN. Fundus autofluorescence patterns in primary intraocular lymphoma. Retina. 2014;34(2):366–72.
24. Ishida T, Ohno-Matsui K, Kaneko Y, Tobita H, Shimada N, Takase H, et al. Fundus autofluorescence patterns in eyes with primary intraocular lymphoma. Retina. 2010;30(1):23–32.
25. Rishi P, Maitra P, Das K, Rishi E, Manchegowda PT. Multimodal imaging characteristics in eyes with vitreoretinal lymphoma treated with intravitreal rituximab. Int Ophthalmol. 2021;41(8):2711–22.
26. Herrlinger U. Primary CNS lymphoma: findings outside the brain. J Neuro-Oncol. 1999;43(3):227–30.
27. Lai J, Chen K, Shi HM, Zhuang L, Zhou X, Xiao JJ, et al. B-scan ultrasound and cytology of the vitreous in primary central nervous system lymphoma with vitreoretinal involvement. Int J Ophthalmol. 2019;12(6):1001–7.
28. Fardeau C, Lee CP, Merle-Béral H, Cassoux N, Bodaghi B, Davi F, et al. Retinal fluorescein, indocyanine green angiography, and optic coherence tomography in non-Hodgkin primary intraocular lymphoma. Am J Ophthalmol. 2009;147(5):886–94, 94.e1.
29. Bowen RC, Raval V, Soto H, Singh AD. Intraocular tumors: angiographic patterns. Asia Pac J Ophthalmol. 2020;9(5):449–60.
30. Wang CC, Carnevale J, Rubenstein JL. Progress in central nervous system lymphomas. Br J Haematol. 2014;166(3):311–25.
31. Wallace DJ, Altemare CR, Shen DF, deSmet MD, Buggage RR, Nussenblatt RB, et al. Primary testicular and intraocular lymphomas: two case reports and a review of the literature. Surv Ophthalmol. 2006;51(1):41–50.
32. Cassoux N, Frenkel S. The importance of cytokines analysis in the diagnosis of vitreoretinal lymphoma. Blood. 2020;98(6):e668–e73.
33. Soussain C, Malaise D. Primary vitreoretinal lymphoma: a diagnostic and management challenge. Blood. 2021;138(17):1519–34.
34. Raja H, Salomão DR, Viswanatha DS, Pulido JS. Prevalence of MYD88 L265P mutation in histologically proven, diffuse large B-cell vitreoretinal lymphoma. Retina. 2016;36(3):624–8.
35. Touitou V, Costopoulos M, Maloum K. Detection of MYD88 mutations in vitreoretinal lymphoma and its implications. JAMA Ophthalmol. 2018;136(10):1104–5.
36. Coupland SE, Foss HD, Hidayat AA, Cockerham GC, Hummel M, Stein H. Extranodal marginal zone B cell lymphomas of the uvea: an analysis of 13 cases. J Pathol. 2002;197(3):333–40.
37. Aronow ME, Portell CA, Sweetenham JW, Singh AD. Uveal lymphoma: clinical features, diagnostic studies, treatment selection, and outcomes. Ophthalmology. 2014;121(1):334–41.

38. Shields CL, Manalac J, Das C, Saktanasate J, Shields JA. Review of spectral domain-enhanced depth imaging optical coherence tomography of tumors of the retina and retinal pigment epithelium in children and adults. Indian J Ophthalmol. 2015;63(2):128–32.
39. Arias JD, Kumar N, Fulco EA, Spaide R, Yannuzzi L, Shields JA, et al. The seasick choroid: a finding on enhanced depth imaging spectral-domain optical coherence tomography of choroidal lymphoma. Retinal Cases Brief Rep. 2013;7(1):19–22.
40. Shields CL, Arepalli S, Pellegrini M, Mashayekhi A, Shields JA. Choroidal lymphoma shows calm, rippled, or undulating topography on enhanced depth imaging optical coherence tomography in 14 eyes. Retina. 2014;34(7):1347–53.

Intraocular Lymphoma: Biopsy Techniques

7

Muhammad Hassan, Michael Heiferman, and Prithvi Mruthyunjaya

Background and Planning

Before pars plana vitrectomy was introduced in the 1970s, enucleation was necessary to make a tissue diagnosis of primary intraocular lymphoma, then known as reticulum cell sarcoma [1–6]. More recently, a revised nomenclature for primary intraocular lymphoma has been suggested as primary central nervous system lymphoma-ophthalmic variant (PCNSL-O) due to similar histological features of the disease. Today, enucleation is reserved for patients with extensive eye disease without any possibility to restore vision or with intractable eye pain. Additionally, with the advancements in surgical techniques and diagnostic testing, such a drastic diagnostic measure is rarely needed. This chapter highlights the procedural tools we have in our armamentarium to help diagnose PCNSL-O.

M. Hassan
Department of Ophthalmology, Byers Eye Institute, Stanford University, Palo Alto, CA, USA
e-mail: hassanm@stanford.edu

M. Heiferman
Department of Ophthalmology and Visual Sciences, Illinois Eye and Ear Infirmary, University of Illinois at Chicago, Chicago, IL, USA
e-mail: mheif@uic.edu

P. Mruthyunjaya (✉)
Stanford Medicine, Palo Alto, CA, USA
e-mail: prithvi9@stanford.edu

A thorough medical history, clinical examination, ophthalmic imaging, and systemic ancillary testing should be performed prior to considering invasive procedures to diagnose PCNSL-O. Often patients with suspected PCNSL-O have failed multiple courses of immunosuppressive or antimicrobial therapy [7]. Additionally, in patients with suspected PCNSL-O, an MRI of the brain and often a high-volume lumbar puncture with cytologic analysis may be performed due to the high incidence of CNS involvement [8–10]. Once CNS involvement has been ruled out, an ocular tissue is often obtained to make the diagnosis.

Intraocular biopsy for the diagnosis of PCNSL-O requires a coordinated approach between multiple teams including ophthalmology, ocular pathology, and medical oncology specializing in lymphoma [11, 12]. A preoperative surgical plan including the biopsy technique, specimens to be obtained, perioperative tissue handling, and tests to be performed should be discussed with the ocular pathologist. The type of biopsy performed is preferred to be the least invasive procedure with the highest diagnostic yield while minimizing ocular morbidity. Some procedures can be both diagnostic and therapeutic and may result in additional tissue specimen due to the therapeutic goal. The biopsy technique chosen directly influences the type, integrity, and amount of the ocular specimen obtained. Since the amount of ocular tissue obtained is relatively small, optimizing the diagnostic yield is critical

V. R. Raval et al. (eds.), *Ocular and Adnexal Lymphoma*, Essentials in Ophthalmology,
https://doi.org/10.1007/978-3-031-24595-4_7

to decrease the need for a repeat surgical procedure. This requires good communication between ophthalmologist, ocular pathologist, surgical, and laboratory staff. The ophthalmologist and ocular pathologist should also work together to involve cytology, microbiology, and send-out laboratory testing as needed.

Vitreous Biopsy

The vitreous is the preferred location for obtaining a tissue specimen in patients with chronic vitritis of unknown etiology, which is partially responsive to immunomodulatory therapy. Vitrectomy can also aid in the diagnosis of PCNSL-O in cases with concurrent CNS disease on imaging but non-diagnostic cerebrospinal fluid analysis [13]. It is important to understand some general principles when planning a surgical approach for the intraocular biopsy of PCNSL-O. It is imperative to have a broad differential in mind as generally these cases are diagnostic challenges with PCNSL-O masquerading as another entity. Therefore, having a differential diagnosis can help tailor the diagnostic testing and help increase the diagnostic yield of the procedure. Furthermore, getting as much undiluted vitreous fluid as safely possible is of key importance. Subsequently, a complete vitrectomy should be performed with the partially diluted vitreous fluid collected. Even though in this chapter, we are highlighting details of both vitreous and chorioretinal biopsy separately, these procedures are not always mutually exclusive. Subretinal aspiration is commonly used to remove deposits from the subretinal space that are visible on examination or guided by intraoperative optical coherence tomography (OCT) imaging. A combination of the two approaches can be performed if the vitreous specimen alone is anticipated to be adequate.

Techniques

The vitreous biopsy technique for patients with suspected PCNSL-O follows a common protocol. A complete core vitrectomy is recommend because cytological analysis is performed along with the frequent addition of molecular testing [14]. In our technique, the procedure begins with the placement of three valved cannulas using a 25-gauge vitrectomy system. An unprimed infusion line is clamped and inserted into the inferotemporal cannula. A 10 cm^3 syringe is connected to the vitrector handpiece allowing for manual aspiration by an assistant (Fig. 7.1a). A cut rate of

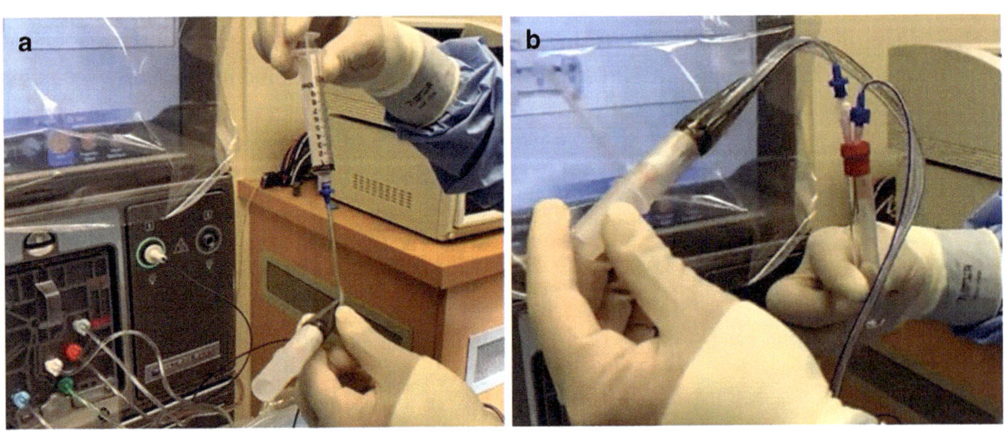

Fig. 7.1 (**a**) Setup showing 10 cm^3 syringe connected to the vitrectomy cutter aspiration line. This will be used by the assistant to aspirate the vitreous. (**b**) Alternative setup with two 18-gauge needles connected to a sterile red top vacutainer for automatic collection of specimens in the collection tubing held vertically by the assistant. Note that the needle with male adapter is attached to vitrectomy probe and the tubing from the other needle extends to the vitrectomy machine

up to 1500 per minute is preferred as higher cut rate may damage potentially viable neoplastic cells. Under wide field visualization through a surgical microscope, the surgeon engages the vitreous cutter while the assistant aspirates 1–2 cm^3 of undiluted vitreous specimen to just avoid globe collapse. It is important to avoid aspiration without cutting vitreous at the cannula to prevent vitreous traction and iatrogenic tears. The goal of this maneuver is to remain in the vitreous with directed removal of visible cellular material. Infusion of air or injection of perfluorocarbon can also be utilized to improve yield of the specimen [15, 16]. An alternative surgeon-controlled aspiration technique has also been published [17, 18]. This technique uses two 18-gauge needles (one connected to a male adapter) that are inserted into a sterile red top BD vacutainer (Becton, Dickinson, and Company, Franklin Lakes, NJ). It is important to make sure that the tube is also sterile on the external surface unlike regular red top blood collection tube. One recommended tube is the 10-mL Draw Red Stopper BD Vacutainer Blood Collection Tube (802012; Becton, Dickinson, and Company, Franklin Lakes, NJ). The other ends of the needles are connected to the aspiration tubing such that the needle with the male adapter receives the tubing from the vitrectomy probe and the tubing from the other needle heads toward the vitrector (Fig. 7.1b). The tube is then held upright by the assistant so that the specimen collects at the bottom of the tube, while the surgeon aspirates the specimen controlling the rate with the foot pedal. It is important to keep the tube upright while suctioning to prevent the specimen from getting drawn up toward the second needle and into the vitrectomy machine. Once the undiluted specimen is collected by any of the techniques described above, the infusion is unclamped to maintain the globe integrity, and a second 10 cm^3 syringe is connected to obtain 8–10 cm^3 of partially diluted vitreous specimen which is commonly used for molecular diagnostic testing. Next, a therapeutic vitrectomy can be performed based on the clinical scenario and surgical plan. The sclerotomies are sutured close at the end of the procedure.

Specimen Division and Processing

It is important to pre-plan the specimen division and processing with the ocular pathologist to ensure rapid processing. This is imperative to avoid lysis of the cells as lymphoma cells begin to deteriorate rapidly once removed from the vitreous cavity [19]. Both undiluted and diluted specimens should be sent for diagnostic testing (details in the next section). Table 7.1 highlights recommended volumes of specimen to be sent for various testing. Additional specimen, if possible, should be collected to increase diagnostic yield of the procedure. The undiluted vitreous specimen should be prioritized for testing specifically for PCNSL-O, while the diluted specimen can also be partially used for the detection of infectious processes (Table 7.2). The vitrector cassette may be included in the final specimen. Once the division of specimen is performed, time is of essence and the vitreous specimens should be hand carried to pathology by either the surgeon or by a reliable team member. However, if immediate transport of the specimen is not possible, then the specimen for cytopathology should be cryopreserved in CytoLyt (Hologic Inc, Santa Clara, CA, USA) solution and the flow cytometry

Table 7.1 Recommended volumes of diluted and undiluted vitreous specimen to be sent for various diagnostic testing

Test	Dilute vitreous specimen (cm^3)	Undilute vitreous specimen (cm^3)
Cytopathology	2–3	0.75–1.0
Flow cytometry	6–8	1.0
MYD 88 PCR		0.2–0.4
Microbiology	0.5	

Table 7.2 Prioritization of dilute and undilute vitreous specimen for various diagnostic testing

Test	Dilute vitreous	Undilute vitreous	Media
Cytopathology	XX	XXX	CytoLyt
Flow cytometry	XXX	XX	RPMI
MYD 88 PCR		XXX	RPMI
Viral PCR	XXX		
Microbiology	XXX	X	

and MYD88 polymerase chain reaction (PCR) specimen should be preserved in the tube containing Roswell Park Memorial Institute (RPMI) culture medium (Table 7.2).

Diagnostic Testing

The specimens collected from the vitrectomy are sent for various tests in addition to cytopathological analysis. These tests may include: (1) immunohistochemistry; (2) flow cytometry; (3), cytokine analysis; (4) PCR for immunoglobulin heavy chain gene (IGH) rearrangement and myeloid differentiation primary response 88 (MYD88) L265P mutation.

Cytopathological identification of malignant lymphoma cells is considered the gold-standard for diagnosing PCNSL-O. The findings seen on cytopathology include atypical cells with large nuclei (2–4 times the normal lymphocytes), coarse chromatin, and high nuclear-cytoplasmic ratio due to scant cytoplasm [20, 21].

Immunohistochemistry analysis for CD20, which is a B-cell biomarker, and CD3, which is a T-cell biomarker, is also used to identify lymphoid cells. Unlike uveitis where T-cell predomination is detected, a higher proportion of B-cells usually supports the diagnosis of B-cell lymphoma [21, 22]. However, T-cell lymphomas can cause PCNSL-O in rare instances.

Flow cytometry is used to assess for monoclonality in cases of suspected lymphoma [23]. This is demonstrated by restriction of the B-cells to kappa and lambda light chain positivity and dominance.

Cytokine analysis for the IL-10 to IL-6 ratio has been shown to reliably distinguish PCNSL-O from inflammatory uveitis [24, 25]. High IL-10 levels are generally seen in PCNSL-O compared to IL-6 which is commonly elevated in uveitis [26, 27]. The absolute values of the interleukins can be affected by dilution of the specimens. Therefore, the ratio of IL-10:IL-6 of greater 1.0 is considered to be suggestive of lymphoma compared to inflammatory uveitis [28]. The ratio of less than 1.0 is labeled as negative and a ratio of 1.0 is considered inconclusive. It is important to note that this ratio does not extend to cases of the less common T-cell lymphomas where the ratio of less than 1.0 is considered positive and greater than 1.0 is considered negative. Overall, IL-10:IL-6 of greater than 1.0 has been found to be positive in 88–92% of cases of PCNSL-O [29, 30]. However, this method alone cannot concretely define PCNSL-O because there is variability in testing kits and techniques between different laboratories. Therefore, most experts use this test as an indirect marker of diagnosis. Additionally, the cytokine levels can be used as a therapeutic marker for measuring response to treatment.

PCR detection of clonal rearrangement of the IGH gene in DNA of the lymphoma cells is another supportive diagnostic test in patients with PCNSL-O [28]. This gene rearrangement is seen in lymphoma cells but was not noted in normal retina and cells from lymphoid hyperplasia [29, 31, 32]. The prevalence of IGH gene rearrangement in cases of PCNSL-O was found to be 80–100%, although false positives are possible when the number of cells is too low [29, 33, 34].

Within the past decade, a specific mutation in the MYD88 gene has been identified as a novel marker for the diagnosis of PCNSL-O. The MYD88 protein is a cell membrane protein that couples with the toll-like receptors involved in recognition of pathogen associated molecular patterns. This activates the innate immune response via nuclear factor (NF-κB) and other cellular cascades [35]. The mutation MYD88-L265P which substitutes leucine with proline at amino acid 256 is a gain in function oncogenically active mutation resulting in increased NF-κB activity promoting cell survival [36]. This mutation was first described in a patient with Waldenstrom's macroglobulinemia. However, this mutation has been commonly associated with various other lymphomas including large B-cells lymphoma of the central nervous system [37, 38]. The presence of this mutation was first noted by Pulido et al. in 2015 and has been found to have a prevalence of 60–80% in cases of PCNSL-O [22, 39, 40]. Additionally, only 5–10 ng DNA is needed to test for this mutation helping with the challenge of the small specimen collection when diagnosing PCSNL-O [41].

Besides these commonly used diagnostic methods, new tests are being studied including targeted next-generation sequencing [22, 28]. Cani et al. utilized next-generation sequencing spanning 126 genes on small volume vitreous specimens from four patients with PCNSL-O [42]. In addition to the MYD88-L265 mutation, they were able to identify multiple new genetic mutations. These include gain of function mutation S243N within MYD88 gene and loss of tumor suppressor gene CDKN2A. The addition of this technology will not only add to our armamentarium of diagnostic testing of PCNSL-O but also provide genetic targets for the development of gene therapies.

Until recently, despite having an array of testing methodologies, there were no uniform guidelines for recommended testing in patients with PNCSL-O. In 2021, a consensus recommendation for the diagnosis of PCNSL-O was published [43]. The study used Delphi methodology with 28 experts in the field to establish these guidelines. In terms of diagnostic testing, performing diagnostic vitrectomy was recommended with the collection of both diluted and undiluted specimen. Testing for IL-10:IL-6 and MYD88 was highly recommended along with cytology, immunophenotyping, and light chain restriction. It was also recommended to use MYD88 and IL10:IL-6 ratio to aid in diagnosis of cases with negative cytology and flow cytometry. However, if MYD88 and IL testing is unavailable, collecting chorioretinal specimen from suspected lesions, or repeat vitrectomy was recommended. Lastly, if there is still high suspicion despite negative ocular testing, a multidisciplinary approach involving neurology and medical oncology may be helpful as the patients may need further CNS evaluation (high-volume LP, serial MRI) and close monitoring of the ocular status to monitor for disease progression.

Diagnostic Yield

Vitreous biopsy specimens may not always result in detection of neoplastic PCNSL-O cells. This is especially common in cases with minimal vitreous findings. This can also happen because the cells may have degenerated due to prolonged time between specimen collection and analysis. The quality of the specimen may also be too poor to perform any cytological or molecular analysis. Therefore, it may be necessary to perform another vitrectomy and collect additional vitreous if there are cells remaining or a chorioretinal biopsy.

Over the years, various studies have demonstrated a range of diagnostic yield (10–99%) of vitreous fluid analysis to help establish a diagnosis of PCNSL-O [21, 44–48]. This wide variation in diagnostic yield may be attributed to major changes in technique and testing strategies over the years. There has been a shift from 20-gauge toward smaller gauge systems for diagnostic vitrectomy. Kanavi et al. compared the yield of their 25-gauge diagnostic vitrectomy against previous studies where 20-gauge vitrectomies are performed and showed improvement in yield in studies where 25-gauge vitrectomy was used [46]. Infusion of air or injection of perfluorocarbon during vitrectomy has been described to increase the yield of undiluted vitreous [15, 49, 50]. However, the change in vitrectomy technique is only one factor responsible for increasing the diagnostic yield of vitreous specimen for diagnosis of PCNSL-O. Testing strategies and methods can cause significant variation in the diagnostic yield.

In studies where cytopathological analysis was mainly used for the diagnosis of PCNSL-O in suspected cases, the diagnostic yield varied between 10% and 50% [44, 45, 47]. The variability in yield has been attributed to the range in pretest probability of suspected lymphoma in the cases analyzed. Notably, lower yields were found in studies that considered patients with other diagnoses in addition to PCNSL-O. Davis et al. were among the first to compare the role of cytological evaluation against the flow cytometry in patients with suspected PCNSL-O and infections [45]. For cases with suspected PCNSL-O, the sensitivity, specificity, positive predictive value (PPV), and negative predictive value (NPV) for cytology were 31%, 100%, 100%, 60.9%, respectively. These results highlight that while a positive cytologic evaluation is certain for the diagnosis of PCNSL-O, a negative result does not always rule out the disease. The additional tests used in the diagnosis of PCNSL-O have variable sensitivities and specificities. The IL-10:IL-6 ratio has been reported to have a sensitivity and specificity ranging between 75% and 99% and 74–85%, respectively [28, 29, 51, 52]. Similarly, IGH gene rearrangements testing has yielded sensitivity between 95% and 100% and specificity between 95% and 99% [22, 29, 52, 53]. A recent meta-analysis by Sehgal et al. reviewed 33 studies during the last decade to calculate the mean along with the coefficient of variation (variation between sensitivity of a particular test across studies) of five commonly used tests in the diagnosis of PCNSL-O [54]. Their results showed that the highest non-weighted mean sensitivities and lowest coefficient of variation were for MYD88 (75% and 0.19) and cytokine analysis (86% and 0.17). Whereas the non-weighted mean sensitivities and coefficient of variation for cytology, flow cytometry, and IGH gene rearrangement studies were 71% (0.39), 58% (0.57), and 66% (0.44), respectively.

It has been shown in multiple studies that combining these diagnostic tests can increase the overall diagnostic yield of the vitreous specimen. In a study by Davis et al., flow cytometry analysis improved the sensitivity (60–94%) and NPV (63–75%), albeit compromising the specificity (60–94%) and PPV (67–88%), depending on which marker was analyzed. Other studies have shown that combining cytology with adjunctive tests can increase the diagnostic yield of vitreous specimen to 66–90%. Yeh et al. showed that adjunctive diagnostic testing (immunohistochemistry, flow cytometry, cytokine evaluation, gene rearrangement studies), when compared to only cytology, increased the diagnostic yield from 25% to 67% [48]. Santos et al. compared various diagnostic statistical parameters for single tests against the combination of two or three tests for diagnosis of PCNSL-O [21]. Their results demonstrated best outcomes when a combination of cytologic smears, immunohistochemistry, and cytokine analysis was utilized to reveal a sensitivity, specificity, PPV, NPV, accuracy, and diagnostic yield of 92%, 98%, 92%, 98%, 96%, and 100%, respectively. Irina et al. demonstrated an increase in sensitivity of vitreous fluid analysis from 62% to 91% and negative predictive value from 86% to 91% by the addition of MYD88 mutation analysis [55]. Therefore, a combination of cytology and additional diagnostic tools can potentially increase the overall efficacy of diagnostic vitrectomy.

Chorioretinal Biopsy

The previously mentioned vitreous biopsy requires malignant lymphoma cells to be present within the vitreous cavity in adequate quantity for diagnosis. However, due to various factors, vitreous biopsy can yield false negative results. These include degeneration or paucity of cells in the vitreous cavity or the specimen obtained. Therefore, it may be necessary to obtain a tissue specimen from the choroid and retina to confirm or rule out a malignant etiology. However, these biopsies are mainly performed when the suspicion for PCNSL-O is high despite a negative vitreous biopsy or in cases of uveal or choroidal lymphomas, as the technique is not without risks. These risks include hemorrhage, endophthalmitis, retinal detachment, proliferative vitreoretinopathy, hypotony, and cataract formation [56]. Like vitreous biopsies, chorioretinal biopsies require proper planning including coordinating care between the ocular surgeon and ocular pathologist. This maximizes yield of the invasive procedure and decreases the rate of unsuccessful attempts.

The surgical technique can be divided into fine-needle aspiration or en-block resection via transscleral or transvitreal approach [57–63]. Fine-needle aspiration is often the procedure of choice; however, one can consider full thickness chorioretinal biopsy if needed. Although tissue collection of infiltrated retina alone is enough for diagnosis, it is common for PCNSL-O to involve the subretinal space, separating the neurosensory retina from the underlying retinal pigment epithelium, which may also be involved. Therefore, it is more ideal to biopsy both retina and choroid to ensure adequate tissue collection for diagnosis. Tumor location, size, or association with adjacent tissue can also guide the chosen approach. Generally, tumors anterior to the equator are approached via transscleral route. This approach is technically easier and has a lower chance of bleeding, retinal detachment, and endophthalmitis. However, there is no direct visualization of the tumor in this method and there is a theoretical risk of extraocular extension. Transvitreal approach, however, is more commonly utilized for tumors posterior to the equator and has the advantage of direct tumor visualization. This method is more technically challenging and is associated with an increased risk of vitreous hemorrhage, retinal detachment, and endophthalmitis. Regardless of the biopsy approach, tissue is often divided into three portions of varying sizes depending on the differential diagnosis: One for histopathological studies, second frozen for immunopathologic and molecular characterization, and third for microorganism cultures.

Techniques

Fine-Needle Aspiration

The lymphoma cells in PCNSL-O are most commonly present in the sub-RPE space. These deposits can be aspirated as part of vitrectomy for vitreous biopsy if visible during the procedure or guided by intraoperative OCT (Fig. 7.2). They are commonly aspirated with a long 27- or 30-gauge needle connected to a 10 mL syringe with a 12–18-inch plastic tubing or via the vitrector using automated aspiration [56, 61–64]. The advantage of using connector tubing is to prevent any movement of the needle, while the assistant performs the aspiration maneuver. The needle can be bent before use to aid in the biopsy of thin lesions. This allows the surgeon to approach the tissue at a flatter angle rather than a 90-degree vertical angle allowing access to a larger area of the lesion while minimizing the risk of perforat-

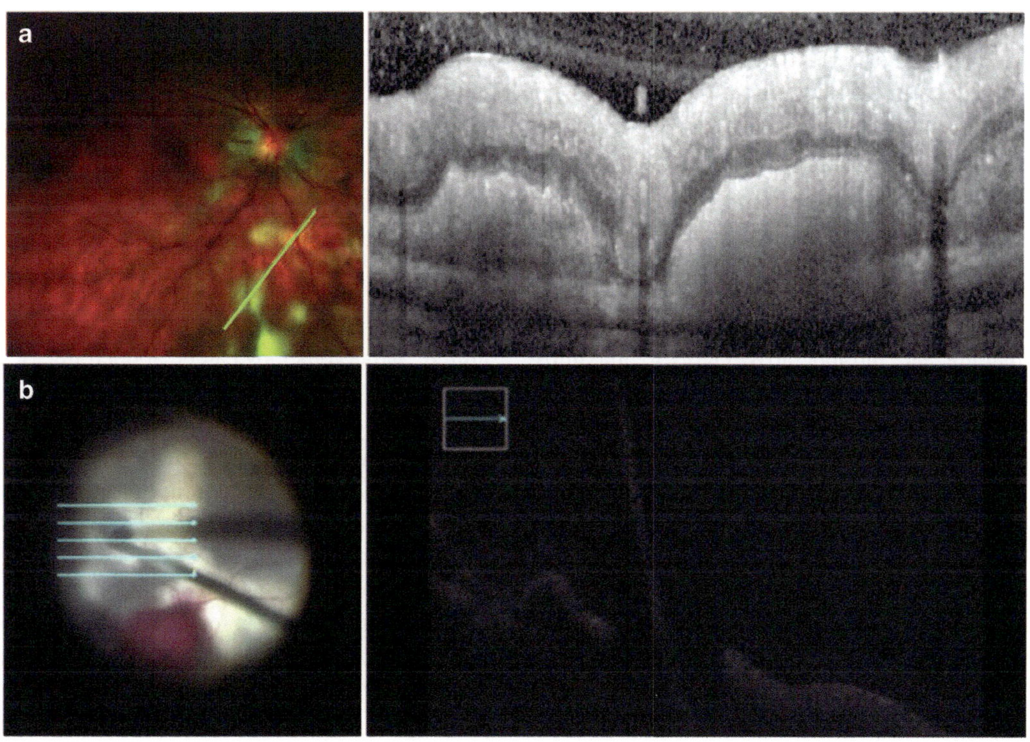

Fig. 7.2 (**a**) Preoperative optical coherence tomography (OCT) scan through suspected primary central nervous system lymphoma-ophthalmic variant (PCNSL-O) demonstrating subretinal infiltrates. (**b**) Intraoperative OCT guided fine-needle aspiration biopsy being performed on a different patient. The needle track is visible on the OCT images. (Courtesy of Sunil Srivastava, MD from Cole Eye Institute)

ing deeper structures. The needle is inserted via the pars plana and advanced until it is within the lesion. Multiple aspirations are performed before carefully withdrawing the needle out of the eye. Although fine-needle aspiration is less invasive than en-block resection, complications including subretinal hemorrhage and choroidal neovascularization have been reported. If vitrectomy is not planned and the location of the tumor is anterior to the equator, fine-needle aspiration to collect the specimen can also be performed via transscleral approach. The area to be biopsied is transilluminated and the biopsy site is marked. A partial thickness scleral pocket is created. A long 27- or 30-gauge needle connected to a 10 mL syringe via 12–18-inch plastic tubing is used to aspirate the specimen. Multiple passes are performed within the pocket created. Once adequate specimen is collected, the pocket is sutured close. Focal retinal detachments can occur in the area of biopsy. Importantly, although least invasive, this method carries a greater risk of inadequate specimen collection.

Transvitreal Chorioretinal Biopsy

The transvitreal approach is another option for obtaining tissue for diagnosis of PCNSL-O [59, 60]. A chorioretinal biopsy is performed using a 23-, 25-, or 27-gauge vitrectomy system and requires careful planning with the ocular pathologist. The biopsy site should be chosen at the edge of the abnormal tissue (guided by preoperative imaging and intraoperative OCT) to maximize the chance of including both active disease and normal tissue for comparison by the pathologist [64, 65]. The most superior edge is preferred to facilitate tamponade and minimize the potential effect of proliferative vitreoretinopathy [66]. Large retinal vessels and subretinal fluid should be avoided to prevent hemorrhage and allow for a single intact chorioretinal specimen. Three valved cannulas are placed at the pars plana in a standard fashion, and a complete vitrectomy is performed. The hyaloid is elevated completely to minimize morbidity in cases that can develop proliferative vitreoretinopathy. An anterior drainage retinotomy may be necessary in cases with exudative retinal detachments at the planned biopsy site. Endolaser or endodiathermy is used to encircle the 1–4 mm^2 biopsy site down to the choroidal vessels with special care to diathermize any involved large retinal vessels (Fig. 7.3a) [67]. The intraocular pressure is raised. A chandelier can be placed to allow for bimanual technique. Multiple instruments can be used to cut the specimen including the vitrector, diamond knife, or vertical scissors that are controlled by hand or a foot pedal (Fig. 7.3b) [68]. Cutting the retina, RPE and choroid usually require multiple passes along with mild posterior pressure. It is often aided by the bimanual use of forceps to provide counter traction on the tissue. A small portion of the specimen should be left uncut to preserve orientation and prevent dislocation. One cannula should be removed and the sclerotomy generously enlarged to remove the specimen. Forceps are passed through the sclerotomy, and the remaining small portion of the specimen is cut [69]. Care is taken to remove both the retinal and choroidal tissue as they may become separated during manipulation (Fig. 7.3c). The infusion is clamped at the time of specimen removal to prevent intraocular turbulence and to avoid the specimen plugging and then projecting from the sclerotomy. The assistant is ready with filter paper adjacent to the sclerotomy over the surgical field. Laser retinopexy is performed around the biopsy site using endolaser. An air-fluid exchange is performed followed by insertion of gas or silicone oil for tamponade. The sclerotomies are sutured, and cryotherapy can be applied in cases concerning for malignancy (Fig. 7.3d).

External Chorioretinal Biopsy

The external approach for chorioretinal biopsy is another method for tissue diagnosis of PCNSL-O [14]. It requires laser photocoagulation of the zone to be biopsied. This can be done in the outpatient setting 1–3 days before surgery if the area of the lesion is clearly visible. Alternatively, in patients with less-than-optimal media clarity, endolaser can be applied during the operative procedure. After complete conjunctival peritomy and isolation of recti muscles, a three port pars plana vitrectomy is performed and vitreous specimen collected as previously explained. After vit-

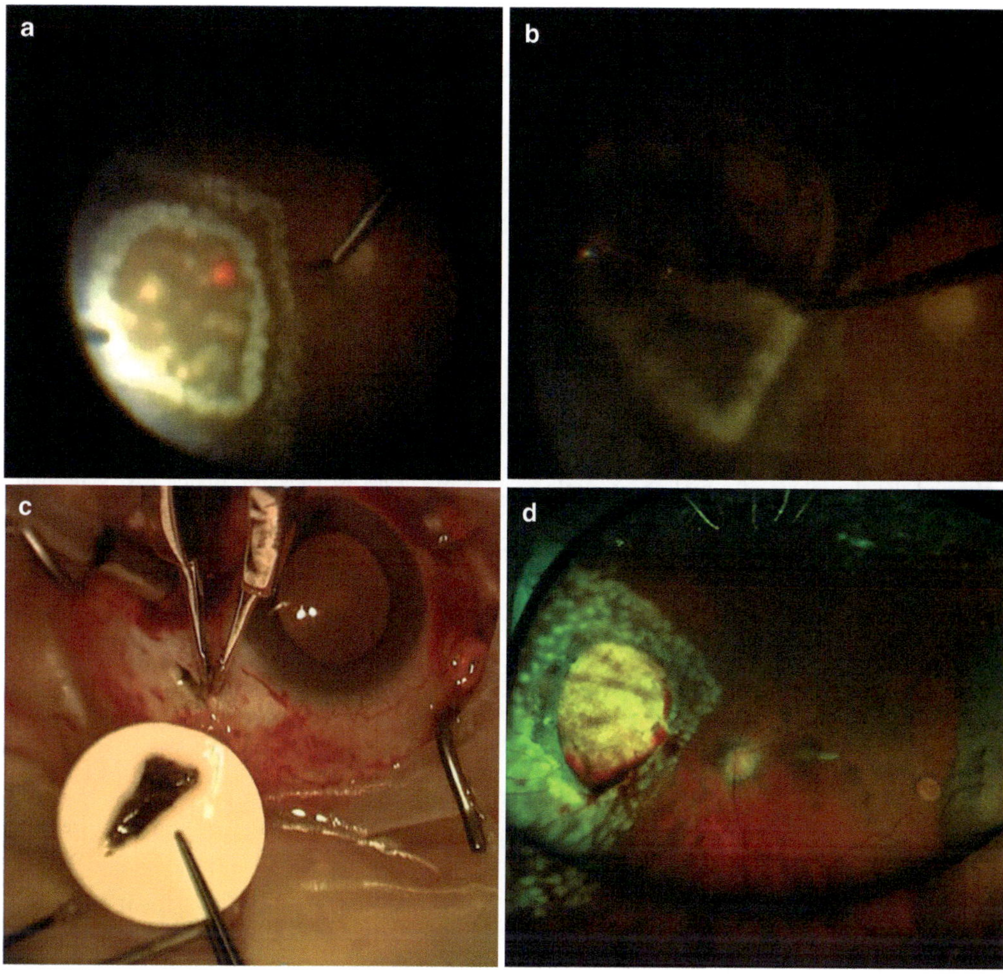

Fig. 7.3 (**a**) Endolaser or endodiathermy is used to encircle the biopsy site down to the choroidal vessels with special care to diathermize any involved large retinal vessels. (**b**) The specimen is cut using the vitrector. Alternate instruments include diamond knife or vertical scissors that are controlled by hand or the foot pedal. (**c**) The specimen is removed by enlarging the sclerotomy and inspected on a white filter paper making sure both retinal and choroidal tissue are obtained. (**d**) Postoperative photograph showing the biopsy site with surrounding laser retinopexy

rectomy, endolaser is introduced and applied to the area to be biopsied if it was not performed preoperatively. The area to be biopsied can be transilluminated and a boundary is marked at the scleral biopsy site. A nearly full thickness hinged scleral flap is created exposing the choroid. A penetrating diathermy is applied through the choroid and retina along the outer margin of the choroidal bed. Two similar sized incisions parallel to the limbus are created and a full thickness edge of the retina and choroid is grasped using 0.12 forceps by passing it through one of the incisions. This is followed by two perpendicular incisions demarcating a block of the chorioretinal tissue, which is removed. It is imperative that the tissue is only grasped with forceps once while these maneuvers are being performed so that tissue architecture remains intact and to avoid crush artifact. The scleral flap is sutured followed by fluid gas exchange and completion of the vitrectomy procedure. This approach provides en-block removal of the area of interest providing excellent anatomical integrity for tissue diagnosis of PCNSL-O.

Diagnostic Yield

As chorioretinal biopsy is often the second choice in cases with inconclusive vitreous biopsy and high suspicion for malignancy due to limited response to therapy or involvement of fellow eye despite treatment, the published literature on the topic is mainly limited to case reports and small case series [12, 56, 60, 66, 70]. Johnston et al. retrospectively reviewed chorioretinal biopsies performed in atypical cases of uveitis [66]. Four patients underwent external chorioretinal biopsies, while ten patients had transvitreal chorioretinal biopsies performed. The biopsies confirmed the diagnosis of a malignant etiology in seven cases and successfully ruled out malignancy in the remaining six cases, although an alternative tissue diagnosis was not confirmed. The complications noted in this series included retinal detachment with subretinal hemorrhage in one patient, cataract progression in one patient, and phthisis in one patient. Another small case series of three patients reported successful identification of underlying etiology in patients who underwent transvitreal chorioretinal biopsies [60]. Mastropasqua et al. recently performed a retrospective review of 29 patients with severe uveitis requiring a chorioretinal biopsy for suspected PCNSL-O [12]. Biopsy was able to provide a tissue diagnosis in 26 cases with 17 cases (56%) testing positive for PCNSL-O and nine cases (31%) with other etiologies were identified. No specific diagnosis was achieved in three cases. Postoperative complications included vitreous hemorrhage and retinal detachment in two patients each.

Based on these studies, chorioretinal biopsies provide an accurate tissue diagnosis and can play a significant role in cases of suspected PCNSL-O, but the procedure is not without risk. More recently, utilization of immunophenotypic and molecular testing along with cytology has improved the diagnostic accuracy of vitreous biopsy for PCNSL-O, reducing the need for chorioretinal tissue sampling.

References

1. Raju VK, Green WR. Reticulum cell sarcoma of the uvea. Ann Ophthalmol. 1982;14(6):555–60.
2. Vogel MH, Font RL, Zimmerman LE, Levine RA. Reticulum cell sarcoma of the retina and uvea. Report of six cases and review of the literature. Am J Ophthalmol. 1968;66(2):205–15.
3. Machemer R, Buettner H, Parel JM. Vitrectomy, a pars plana approach. Instrumentation. Mod Probl Ophthalmol. 1972;10:172–7.
4. Machemer R, Buettner H, Norton EW, Parel JM. Vitrectomy: a pars plana approach. Trans Am Acad Ophthalmol Otolaryngol. 1971;75(4):813–20.
5. Machemer R, Norton EW. Vitrectomy, a pars plana approach. II. Clinical experience. Mod Probl Ophthalmol. 1972;10:178–85.
6. Machemer R, Parel JM, Norton EW. Vitrectomy: a pars plana approach. Technical improvements and further results. Trans Am Acad Ophthalmol Otolaryngol. 1972;76(2):462–6.
7. Amaro MH, Muccioli C, Abreu MT. Ocular masquerade syndrome due to intraocular lymphoma--two forms of retinal pigment epithelium involvement: case reports. Arq Bras Oftalmol. 2007;70(3):521–5.
8. Zhuang L, Lai J, Chen K, Ding T, Yuan Y, Ma Y, et al. Intraocular involvement is associated with a high risk of disease relapse in primary central nervous system lymphoma. Oncol Rep. 2019;41(1):397–404.
9. Rockwood EJ, Zakov ZN, Bay JW. Combined malignant lymphoma of the eye and CNS (reticulum-cell sarcoma). Report of three cases. J Neurosurg. 1984;61(2):369–74.
10. Baehring JM, Androudi S, Longtine JJ, Betensky RA, Sklar J, Foster CS, et al. Analysis of clonal immunoglobulin heavy chain rearrangements in ocular lymphoma. Cancer. 2005;104(3):591–7.
11. Zhou HP, Tanaka R, Kaburaki T. Multidisciplinary diagnostic approach in intraocular lymphoma featuring pseudo-hypopyon: case series and literature review. Ocul Immunol Inflamm. 2021;29(3):490–5.
12. Mastropasqua R, Thaung C, Pavesio C, Lightman S, Westcott M, Okhravi N, et al. The role of chorioretinal biopsy in the diagnosis of intraocular lymphoma. Am J Ophthalmol. 2015;160(6):1127–32.e1.
13. Parver LM, Font RL. Malignant lymphoma of the retina and brain. Initial diagnosis by cytologic examination of vitreous aspirate. Arch Ophthalmol. 1979;97(8):1505–7.
14. Gonzales JA, Chan CC. Biopsy techniques and yields in diagnosing primary intraocular lymphoma. Int Ophthalmol. 2007;27(4):241–50.
15. Zhao M, Yu Y, Liu W. Vitreous biopsy under air: technique, complications, and volume outcomes. Ophthalmic Surg Lasers Imaging Retina. 2019;50(6):365–70.

16. Tang PH, Karkhur S, Nguyen QD. Obtaining undiluted vitreous sample using small gauge pars plana vitrectomy and air infusion. Am J Ophthalmol Case Rep. 2020;19:100768.
17. Malinowski SM. The vitreous trap: a simple, surgeon-controlled technique for obtaining undiluted vitreous and subretinal specimens during pars plana vitrectomy. Retina. 2010;30(5):828–9.
18. Moshfeghi AA, Albini TA, Kitchens JW, Leng T, Moshfeghi DM. The vitreous trap: a simple, surgeon-controlled technique for obtaining undiluted vitreous and subretinal specimens during pars plana vitrectomy. Retina. 2011;31(2):426–7; author reply 7.
19. Whitcup SM, Chan CC, Buggage RR, Nussenblatt RB, Byrnes GA, Rubin BI. Improving the diagnostic yield of vitrectomy for intraocular lymphoma. Arch Ophthalmol. 2000;118(3):446.
20. Chan CC, Rubenstein JL, Coupland SE, Davis JL, Harbour JW, Johnston PB, et al. Primary vitreoretinal lymphoma: a report from an International Primary Central Nervous System Lymphoma Collaborative Group symposium. Oncologist. 2011;16(11):1589–99.
21. Santos MC, Jiang A, Li AS, Rao PK, Wilson B, Harocopos GJ. Vitreoretinal lymphoma: optimizing diagnostic yield and accuracy. Am J Ophthalmol. 2021;236:120–9.
22. Pulido JS, Johnston PB, Nowakowski GS, Castellino A, Raja H. The diagnosis and treatment of primary vitreoretinal lymphoma: a review. Int J Retina Vitreous. 2018;4:18.
23. Cho BJ, Kim DY, Park UC, Lee JY, Yoon YH, Yu HG. Clinical features and treatment outcomes of vitreoretinal lymphoma according to its association with CNS lymphoma. Ocul Immunol Inflamm. 2018;26(3):365–71.
24. Fisson S, Ouakrim H, Touitou V, Baudet S, Ben Abdelwahed R, Donnou S, et al. Cytokine profile in human eyes: contribution of a new cytokine combination for differential diagnosis between intraocular lymphoma or uveitis. PLoS One. 2013;8(2):e52385.
25. Caraballo JN, Snyder MR, Johnston PB, Neill BPO, Raja H, Balsanek JG, et al. Vitreoretinal lymphoma versus uveitis: cytokine profile and correlations. Ocul Immunol Inflamm. 2014;22(1):34–41.
26. Gupta M, Han JJ, Stenson M, Maurer M, Wellik L, Hu G, et al. Elevated serum IL-10 levels in diffuse large B-cell lymphoma: a mechanism of aberrant JAK2 activation. Blood. 2012;119(12):2844–53.
27. Cassoux N, Giron A, Bodaghi B, Tran TH, Baudet S, Davy F, et al. IL-10 measurement in aqueous humor for screening patients with suspicion of primary intraocular lymphoma. Invest Ophthalmol Vis Sci. 2007;48(7):3253–9.
28. Dawson AC, Williams KA, Appukuttan B, Smith JR. Emerging diagnostic tests for vitreoretinal lymphoma: a review. Clin Exp Ophthalmol. 2018;46(8):945–54.
29. Kimura K, Usui Y, Goto H, Japanese Intraocular Lymphoma Study G. Clinical features and diagnostic significance of the intraocular fluid of 217 patients with intraocular lymphoma. Jpn J Ophthalmol. 2012;56(4):383–9.
30. Costopoulos M, Touitou V, Golmard JL, Darugar A, Fisson S, Bonnemye P, et al. ISOLD: a new highly sensitive interleukin score for intraocular lymphoma diagnosis. Ophthalmology. 2016;123(7):1626–8.
31. Shen DF, Zhuang Z, LeHoang P, Boni R, Zheng S, Nussenblatt RB, et al. Utility of microdissection and polymerase chain reaction for the detection of immunoglobulin gene rearrangement and translocation in primary intraocular lymphoma. Ophthalmology. 1998;105(9):1664–9.
32. Chan CC. Molecular pathology of primary intraocular lymphoma. Trans Am Ophthalmol Soc. 2003;101:275–92.
33. Coupland SE, Hummel M, Muller HH, Stein H. Molecular analysis of immunoglobulin genes in primary intraocular lymphoma. Invest Ophthalmol Vis Sci. 2005;46(10):3507–14.
34. Coupland SE, Perez-Canto A, Hummel M, Stein H, Heimann H. Assessment of HOPE fixation in vitrectomy specimens in patients with chronic bilateral uveitis (masquerade syndrome). Graefes Arch Clin Exp Ophthalmol. 2005;243(9):847–52.
35. Deguine J, Barton GM. MyD88: a central player in innate immune signaling. F1000Prime Rep. 2014;6:97.
36. Ngo VN, Young RM, Schmitz R, Jhavar S, Xiao W, Lim KH, et al. Oncogenically active MYD88 mutations in human lymphoma. Nature. 2011;470(7332):115–9.
37. Bruno A, Boisselier B, Labreche K, Marie Y, Polivka M, Jouvet A, et al. Mutational analysis of primary central nervous system lymphoma. Oncotarget. 2014;5(13):5065–75.
38. Gonzalez-Aguilar A, Idbaih A, Boisselier B, Habbita N, Rossetto M, Laurenge A, et al. Recurrent mutations of MYD88 and TBL1XR1 in primary central nervous system lymphomas. Clin Cancer Res. 2012;18(19):5203–11.
39. Pulido JS, Salomao DR, Frederick LA, Viswanatha DS. MyD-88 L265P mutations are present in some cases of vitreoretinal lymphoma. Retina. 2015;35(4):624–7.
40. Raja H, Salomao DR, Viswanatha DS, Pulido JS. Prevalence of Myd88 L265p mutation in histologically proven, diffuse large B-cell vitreoretinal lymphoma. Retina. 2016;36(3):624–8.
41. Pulido JS, Raja H, Vile RG, Salomao DR, Viswanatha DS. Mighty MyD88 in health and disease. Retina. 2016;36(3):429–31.
42. Cani AK, Hovelson DH, Demirci H, Johnson MW, Tomlins SA, Rao RC. Next generation sequencing of vitreoretinal lymphomas from small-volume intraocular liquid biopsies: new routes to targeted therapies. Oncotarget. 2017;8(5):7989–98.

43. Carbonell D, Mahajan S, Chee SP, Sobolewska B, Agrawal R, Bulow T, et al. Consensus recommendations for the diagnosis of vitreoretinal lymphoma. Ocul Immunol Inflamm. 2021;29(3):507–20.
44. Akpek EK, Ahmed I, Hochberg FH, Soheilian M, Dryja TP, Jakobiec FA, et al. Intraocular-central nervous system lymphoma: clinical features, diagnosis, and outcomes. Ophthalmology. 1999;106(9):1805–10.
45. Davis JL, Miller DM, Ruiz P. Diagnostic testing of vitrectomy specimens. Am J Ophthalmol. 2005;140(5):822–9.
46. Kanavi MR, Soheilian M, Hosseini SB, Azari AA. 25-Gauge transconjunctival diagnostic vitrectomy in suspected cases of intraocular lymphoma: a case series and review of the literature. Int J Ophthalmol. 2014;7(3):577–81.
47. Mruthyunjaya P, Jumper JM, McCallum R, Patel DJ, Cox TA, Jaffe GJ. Diagnostic yield of vitrectomy in eyes with suspected posterior segment infection or malignancy. Ophthalmology. 2002;109(6):1123–9.
48. Yeh S, Weichel ED, Faia LJ, Albini TA, Wroblewski KK, Stetler-Stevenson M, et al. 25-Gauge transconjunctival sutureless vitrectomy for the diagnosis of intraocular lymphoma. Br J Ophthalmol. 2010;94(5):633–8.
49. Quiroz-Mercado H, Rivera-Sempertegui J, Macky TA, Navarro-Lopez P, Griselda-Alvarez L, Ibarra-Ponce N, et al. Performing vitreous biopsy by perfluorocarbon-perfused vitrectomy. Am J Ophthalmol. 2005;140(6):1161–3.
50. Gariano RF. Vitreous biopsy with air infusion: safety and effectiveness. Retina. 2000;20(4):422–3.
51. Lobo A, Okhravi N, Adamson P, Clark BJ, Lightman S. Protocol for the use of polymerase chain reaction in the detection of intraocular large B-cell lymphoma in ocular samples. J Mol Diagn. 2007;9(1):113–21.
52. Wang Y, Shen D, Wang VM, Sen HN, Chan CC. Molecular biomarkers for the diagnosis of primary vitreoretinal lymphoma. Int J Mol Sci. 2011;12(9):5684–97.
53. Sugita S, Takase H, Sugamoto Y, Arai A, Miura O, Mochizuki M. Diagnosis of intraocular lymphoma by polymerase chain reaction analysis and cytokine profiling of the vitreous fluid. Jpn J Ophthalmol. 2009;53(3):209–14.
54. Sehgal A, Pulido JS, Mashayekhi A, Milman T, Deak GG. Diagnosing vitreoretinal lymphomas-an analysis of the sensitivity of existing tools. Cancers. 2022;14(3):598.
55. Bonzheim I, Giese S, Deuter C, Susskind D, Zierhut M, Waizel M, et al. High frequency of MYD88 mutations in vitreoretinal B-cell lymphoma: a valuable tool to improve diagnostic yield of vitreous aspirates. Blood. 2015;126(1):76–9.
56. Mastropasqua R, Di Carlo E, Sorrentino C, Mariotti C, da Cruz L. Intraocular biopsy and immunomolecular pathology for "unmasking" intraocular inflammatory diseases. J Clin Med. 2019;8(10):1733.
57. Peyman GA, Juarez CP, Raichand M. Full-thickness eye-wall biopsy: long-term results in 9 patients. Br J Ophthalmol. 1981;65(10):723–6.
58. Peyman GA, Meisels HI, Batko KA, Vlchek JK. Full-thickness eye wall biopsy. I. An experimental approach to the tissue diagnosis and study of choroidal and retinal lesions. Investig Ophthalmol. 1975;14(6):484–7.
59. Nussenblatt RB, Davis JL, Palestine AG. Chorioretinal biopsy for diagnostic purposes in cases of intraocular inflammatory disease. Dev Ophthalmol. 1992;23:133–8.
60. Cassoux N, Charlotte F, Rao NA, Bodaghi B, Merle-Beral H, Lehoang P. Endoretinal biopsy in establishing the diagnosis of uveitis: a clinicopathologic report of three cases. Ocul Immunol Inflamm. 2005;13(1):79–83.
61. Eide N, Walaas L. Fine-needle aspiration biopsy and other biopsies in suspected intraocular malignant disease: a review. Acta Ophthalmol. 2009;87(6):588–601.
62. Westerfeld C, Mukai S. Retinal and choroidal biopsy. Int Ophthalmol Clin. 2009;49(1):145–54.
63. Sarafzadeh S, Correa ZM, Dhamija A, Augsburger JJ, Trichopoulos N. Intraocular lymphoma diagnosed by fine-needle aspiration biopsy. Acta Ophthalmol. 2010;88(6):705–10.
64. Kumar JB, Ehlers JP, Sharma S, Srivastava SK. Intraoperative OCT for uveitis-related vitreoretinal surgery in the DISCOVER study. Ophthalmol Retina. 2018;2(10):1041–9.
65. Rutzen AR, Ortega-Larrocea G, Dugel PU, Chong LP, Lopez PF, Smith RE, et al. Clinicopathologic study of retinal and choroidal biopsies in intraocular inflammation. Am J Ophthalmol. 1995;119(5):597–611.
66. Johnston RL, Tufail A, Lightman S, Luthert PJ, Pavesio CE, Cooling RJ, et al. Retinal and choroidal biopsies are helpful in unclear uveitis of suspected infectious or malignant origin. Ophthalmology. 2004;111(3):522–8.
67. Cole CJ, Kwan AS, Laidlaw DA, Aylward GW. A new technique of combined retinal and choroidal biopsy. Br J Ophthalmol. 2008;92(10):1357–60.
68. Char DH, Kemlitz AE, Miller T. Intraocular biopsy. Ophthalmol Clin N Am. 2005;18(1):177–85, x.
69. Kvanta A, Seregard S, Kopp ED, All-Ericsson C, Landau I, Berglin L. Choroidal biopsies for intraocular tumors of indeterminate origin. Am J Ophthalmol. 2005;140(6):1002–6.
70. Lim LL, Suhler EB, Rosenbaum JT, Wilson DJ. The role of choroidal and retinal biopsies in the diagnosis and management of atypical presentations of uveitis. Trans Am Ophthalmol Soc. 2005;103:84–91; discussion 92.

Vitreoretinal Lymphoma: Intraocular Therapy

8

Jacob Pe'er and Shahar Frenkel

Introduction

PCNSL-O is the most common lymphoma affecting the eye and its surroundings. Still, it is a rare malignancy that almost always involves the vitreous and may additionally involve the retina, subretinal space, retinal pigment epithelium, and the optic nerve [1]. These are high-grade, mostly B-cell malignancies that are associated with a poor prognosis if the patient also develops central nervous system lymphoma (CNSL) [2]. T-cell PCNSL-Os are much less common, constituting only about 10% of the cases [1, 3]. Three other groups of intraocular lymphomas involve various parts of the uvea and are usually low-grade B-cell lymphomas [2].

PCNSL-O is often associated with CNSL and is considered by specialists as a subgroup of CNSL [4, 5], and 9% of the patients initially diagnosed with either PCNSL-O or CNSL are simultaneously diagnosed with lymphoma at the other site as well [1]. It has been reported that 56–90% of PCNSL-O patients ultimately develop CNSL, while 11–54% of patients with CNSL develop PCNSL-O [1, 4, 6–9]. PCNSL-O is commonly diagnosed in patients over 50 years of age, although younger patients are also diagnosed. There is no clear sex predilection [4, 5], although in several studies, more women were affected than men [1, 10, 11].

The hallmark of PCNSL-O is the presence of cells in the vitreous, mainly in clumps, which is often misdiagnosed as non-responsive uveitis, along with retinal and subretinal infiltrates [12]. In contrast with the reduction in visual acuity in uveitis with similar findings, the visual acuity of PCNSL-O patients is unexpectedly good.

A clinical diagnosis of PCNSL-O often relies on the above-mentioned clinical findings, sometimes assisted by neurological symptoms and CNS MRI findings. However, a biopsy is needed to confirm the diagnosis. Some experts find that a suggestive clinical picture of PCNSL-O with a positive brain biopsy for CNSL is sufficient for the diagnosis of PCNSL-O. Usually, one performs a diagnostic vitrectomy or vitreous tap without or with an anterior chamber tap. The vitreous samples can be analyzed for the presence of malignant cells by cytopathology with possible immunohistochemical staining or flow cytometry to identify the cell type and monoclonality. Other diagnostic methods are the measurement of the levels of interleukins (IL-10 and IL-6) and the ratio between them, which was found to be a very sensitive test, also in aqueous humor samples from the anterior chamber (AC) of the eye; PCR for detection of immunoglobulin

J. Pe'er (✉) · S. Frenkel
Ocular Oncology Service, Division of Ophthalmology, Hadassah – Hebrew University Medical Center, Jerusalem, Israel
e-mail: peer@hadassah.org.il; Shahar@hadassah.org.il

V. R. Raval et al. (eds.), *Ocular and Adnexal Lymphoma*, Essentials in Ophthalmology,
https://doi.org/10.1007/978-3-031-24595-4_8

heavy chain (IgH) or T-cell receptor (TCR) gene rearrangement which indicates clonality of malignant cells; and a search for an L265P mutation in the myeloid differentiation primary response gene 88 (MYD88) in diffuse large B-cell lymphoma [4, 9, 13–17].

Since intraocular lymphoma was first recognized in 1951 [18, 19], initially as ocular reticulum cell sarcoma, its treatment has evolved from enucleation [19] through radiation therapy, with or without whole-brain radiotherapy, systemic chemotherapy, intrathecal chemotherapy, intravitreal chemotherapy, and biological therapy. All of these modalities have been successful in eradicating intraocular disease.

Failing to treat the eyes will result in blindness, but failing to treat the brain would result in death. There is a years-long debate whether adding systemic treatment to PCNSL-O patients with no clear sign of CNSL can prevent CNSL [4]. So far, there have been no randomized clinical trials that can lead to a consensus recommendation that will solve this debate. In their report, the International CNSL Collaborative Group recommended systemic treatment if the disease involves the CNS and local ocular treatment if the disease involves only the eye, with close follow-up and ongoing collaboration between neuro-oncologists and ophthalmologists [4]. Several other studies presented additional data to support that recommendation [9, 11, 20–23].

Radiation therapy in doses ranging between 30 and 50 Gy was the gold standard for treating intraocular lymphoma in many institutions. However, because of a high recurrence rate and ocular complications, radiation is less often considered nowadays for therapy of PCNSL-O [8]. Systemic chemotherapy, mainly with high-dose methotrexate (MTX), sometimes combined with rituximab, which is used for treating CNSL, has also been used for treating PCNSL-O. However, the limited penetration of systemic drugs into the vitreous is well known, leading to incomplete response [8]. Therefore, direct intravitreal injection of drugs, including, among others, chemotherapeutic and biological drugs, has become routine in the treatment of various infectious, inflammatory, neovascular, and malignant intraocular diseases. Intravitreal chemotherapy has become the most common method of treating PCNSL-O. In this chapter, we review the current status of intraocular chemotherapy for PCNSL-O.

Intravitreal Chemotherapy

Intravitreal chemotherapy can be given as primary therapy for PCNSL-O or as adjuvant therapy to other treatment methods, although in recent years, the primary intravitreal treatment has become the gold standard.

One of the goals of treating cancer is the localized delivery of therapeutics to the cancer without affecting the rest of the body. Intravitreal injections are therefore an ideal delivery route for treating intraocular malignancies. Ericson and associates [24] had performed trials of intravitreal injections of thiotepa, nitrogen mustard, cyclophosphamide, and methotrexate into rabbits' eyes, finding no significant intraocular toxicity except in those treated with nitrogen mustard. They even treated several patients with retinoblastoma with intravitreal injections of thiotepa [25]. From 1961 to 1995, it took three decades for another attempt with an intravitreal treatment for retinoblastoma [26]. However, shortly thereafter (1996) intravitreal melphalan for retinoblastoma became a routine practice in Japan [27, 28], while intravitreal methotrexate (MTX) was suggested for the treatment of PCNSL-O in 1997 [29].

In the following paragraphs, we will describe the main drugs currently used in intravitreal injections for treating PCNSL-O.

Intravitreal Methotrexate

Methotrexate (MTX) is currently the most commonly used drug for PCNSL-O. MTX is an antimetabolite that acts by competitive inhibition of the enzyme dihydrofolate reductase, resulting in reduced thymine synthesis, an essential nuclear base in DNA [30].

Fishburne and associates at the Oregon Health & Science University (OHSU, Portland, Oregon, USA) [29] were the first to report in 1997 on the treatment of PCNSL-O in seven eyes of four patients with intravitreal injections of 400 μg of MTX, injecting 6–11 injections per eye, in conjunction with systemic chemotherapy delivered by hyper-osmotic blood–brain barrier disruption (BBBD). All patients had complete remission without serious ocular toxic effects.

These promising results were repeated by de Smet and associates [22, 23, 31, 32] from the National Eye Institute at the NIH, who reported two successful cases of treating recurrent PCNSL-O with combined intravitreal chemotherapy, one case with intravitreal MTX and thiotepa and one case with intravitreal MTX and dexamethasone, with a full remission.

Following the clinical results, they set out to test the pharmacokinetics of a single dose of intraocular injection of MTX in a blind eye of a patient with recurrent PCNSL-O. Injecting 400 μg resulted in lymphocytotoxic concentrations for 5 days [31]. Next, Velez and associates [33] investigated the pharmacokinetics and toxicity of several intravitreal injections of 400 μg MTX in rabbits' eyes, together with single injections of fluorouracil and dexamethasone. They found that MTX vitreous levels remain therapeutic (>0.5 μM) in the rabbit eye for 48–72 h without evidence of toxicity.

In 2002 the OHSU group together with the Hadassah Medical Center group reported a larger series of 26 eyes of 16 HIV-negative patients with PCNSL-O from the two centers, treated by intravitreal injections of 400 μg MTX in 0.1 mL [34]. Their protocol included three phases: two injections per week for a month as an induction phase; weekly injection for a month in one center and 2 months in the other center as consolidation phase; and subsequently a maintenance phase of monthly injections to complete a year of treatment. All eyes achieved remission after a maximum of 12 MTX injections (mean of 8.5 injections). Three patients of the center with the shorter consolidation phase had a relapse in the eye and were treated again using the same intravitreal injections protocol with complete remission. Unfortunately, six of the 16 patients died in follow-up as a result of progressive CNSL, but without clinical ocular involvement.

Frenkel and associates at the Hadassah Medical Center (HMC) reported a large series of 44 eyes of 26 patients from a single center, who were treated by the same induction-consolidation-maintenance regimen of intravitreal MTX injections [35] (this group included half of the patients reported by Smith et al. [34]). This HMC group of patients also included several patients with T-cell lymphoma [35]. Clinical remission was reached in all eyes after an average of 6.4 injections, with 95% of the eyes needing 13 injections or less to be cleared of lymphoma cells. None of the patients had a relapse. All patients in these reports who had PCNSL-CNS were also treated for the brain disease by systemic chemotherapy. Sou and colleagues [36] reported similar results in one Japanese center.

The most common side effects of the intravitreal injections are conjunctival hyperemia and transient keratopathy, ranging from diffuse punctate keratopathy to severe epitheliopathy, which usually subside during the maintenance phase [1, 34, 37]. Keratopathy usually leads to a transient decrease in the visual acuity, sometimes even more than expected to that degree of dryness, which usually improves after completion of the consolidation phase. Other complications are acceleration of existing cataract, which could also be due to diagnostic vitrectomy, neovascular glaucoma, which could have occurred because of the PCNSL-O itself, and sterile intraocular inflammation that can be successfully treated by corticosteroids [1, 34, 38]. Patients treated with BBBD for CNSL may develop maculopathy without a significant effect on their visual acuity [34]. None of the patients who were treated with intravitreal injections of MTX but were not treated with BBBD developed maculopathy [39].

There have been some differences in the protocols used in various institutions for intravitreal MTX monotherapy for treating PCNSL-O. Most treating ophthalmologists inject 400 μg in 0.1 mL, as in the first studies. Only a few injected less than 400 μg, and some, like us, reduced the injection volume to 0.05 mL. However, the number of injections varies widely, and some will inject "according to the clinical behavior of the lymphoma" [40]. Reducing the number of injections, especially in the induction and consolidation phase, was attempted to reduce the rate and severity of the keratopathy. However, shorter induction and consolidation phases increased the local recurrence rate from 2.5% [1] to 18–33% [41, 42].

Combined intravitreal injections with systemic chemotherapy, mostly high-dose MTX, have been used in treating PCNSL-O [40–43]. However, there is no evidence that the systemic MTX improves or shortens the time of treatment or increases the time to relapse and progression of the PCNSL-O. In addition, there is no proof that systemic chemotherapy prevents the development of CNSL in PCNSL-O patients without CNSL [9, 11, 20–23]. In our experience and that of others, intravitreal MTX injections should be used for treating PCNSL-O and systemic chemotherapy for treating PCNSL-CNS. We recommend avoiding systemic chemotherapy in the treatment of PCNSL-O patients when CNS is not involved. Other combination treatments for PCNSL-O are the use of intravitreal MTX and rituximab, sometimes with the addition of systemic chemotherapy or even radiotherapy [21, 44–46].

Intravitreal Rituximab

Rituximab is a humanized monoclonal antibody that targets CD20-positive B-cells in all stages, from a pre-B-cell through a mature B-cell. Thus, CD20 also presents on lymphomatous B-cells in PCNSL-O and CNSL. Rituximab was approved in 1997 by the FDA to be used in B-cell lymphomas of various types. With the vast majority of PCNSL-O and CNSL resulting from malignant B-cells, rituximab seems an ideal, specific drug for intravitreal therapy. The hope was to reach the same tumoricidal effect with milder side effects and fewer injections than the full MTX protocol. Unfortunately, this treatment cannot help the minority of T-cell PCNSL-O patients.

In contrast to the clinical data first and preclinical data later we have seen above for intravitreal melphalan for retinoblastoma and intravitreal MTX for PCNSL-O, Intravitreal rituximab was first tested in animal studies. All these studies tested injection of 1 mg/0.1 mL rituximab. Kim and associates [47], investigating the pharmacokinetics of intravitreal injections of rituximab into rabbit eyes, found a half-life of 4.7 days in both the aqueous and vitreous. Pulido and colleagues [48] found that rituximab penetrated all retinal layers in rabbit eyes, and Kitzmann and associates [49] showed no toxicity to the rabbit eyes. Mineo and colleagues [50] showed eradication of lymphoma in more than half of the animals and significant inhibition of tumor progression in the rest.

Kitzmann and colleagues [49] were the first to report their experience with intravitreal injections of rituximab in treating five eyes of three patients in 2007. They used 3–4 injections of 1 mg/0.1 mL rituximab with a good response, no toxicity, and no evidence of recurrence after a short median follow-up of 3.6 months. Ohguro and associates [51] treated two patients who had PCNSL-O relapse after intravitreal MTX by four weekly injections of 1 mg/0.1 mL rituximab with complete remission and no recurrence after 2 months.

Hashida and associates [52] reported their experience in treating 20 eyes of 13 patients who had discontinued previous intravitreal MTX treatment because of severe corneal epitheliopathy. They used four weekly injections of 1 mg/mL rituximab as a one-course protocol, and additional injections were administered when PCNSL-O recurred in 11 of the eyes. All patients completed 1-year follow-up. Twelve eyes showed transient intraocular pressure elevation. No other significant side effects developed.

In 2014 Larkin and associates [53] presented what is still the largest series of intravitreal rituximab-based treatments for treating PCNSL-O, including 48 eyes of 34 patients in clinics in five countries. The eyes were treated with a median of 3.5 injections; the most common interval was monthly. About two-thirds of the eyes were also injected with MTX, usually on the same day with rituximab. Others were treated with more extensive cytotoxic therapies. Complete remission was achieved in 65% of the eyes, and 23% showed partial remission. Among eyes that were treated only by intraocular chemotherapy, 53% experienced complete remission and 11 partial remissions. However, after a median follow-up of 18 months, PCNSL-O recurred in 23% of the eyes. The main complication in this series was cataract in 19% of eyes.

The use of intravitreal rituximab for PCNSL-O was also reported in other small series and case reports. It was used mainly as a secondary treatment [54–56] or in combination with other drugs, mainly MTX [21, 44–46]. Unpublished reports from some centers which were discussed in international meetings indicate that fewer than 6 monthly injections are insufficient to prevent local recurrences, and we urge those with experience to publish their results. There is still no significant series of eyes with PCNSL-O treated by rituximab alone as primary treatment. Such a study should be considered.

Other Drugs for Intravitreal Chemotherapy

The experience with using drugs other than MTX and rituximab for the treatment of PCNSL-O is very limited.

Intravitreal injections of **melphalan** have been often used in recent years for treating retinoblastoma. Melphalan is a phenylalanine derivative of nitrogen mustard and an alkylating agent. Shields and associates [57] reported in 2017 their experience in treating three eyes of two patients with PCNSL-O by intravitreal injections of 10 μg/0.1 mL melphalan. One of the patients with bilateral PCNSL-O showed clinical remission within 3 weeks after a single injection. Recurrence in one of the eyes was treated by additional six bimonthly injections with a good response and no recurrence after 19 months of follow-up. The other patient with bilateral PCNSL-O was treated by intravitreal melphalan in one eye and MTX in the other eye. The PCNSL-O in the eye treated with melphalan was cured by one injection. No toxicity was observed. This group expanded their use of melphalan and reported on 12 more patients with encouraging results [20]. Damato and associates [58] reported their good experience with intravitreal melphalan in treating a single patient with PCNSL-O.

Thiotepa is an organophosphorus alkylating agent, which results in crosslinking of the double-stranded DNA helix and interferes with DNA replication. Ericson and associates reported their results of using intravitreal thiotepa injections for treating intraocular retinoblastoma in 1961 [25] and tested it in rabbits' eyes in 1964 [24], finding no significant toxicity. de Smet and associates [31, 32] combined thiotepa (2 mg/0.1 mL) with MTX injections in treating a patient with PCNSL-O. However, the thiotepa injection was associated with elevated intraocular pressure and loss of vision. In light of the good results with intravitreal MTX alone, thiotepa is no longer being used.

Corticosteroids have lymphocytotoxic effect; however, the response is usually partial with a high local recurrence rate once the steroids are discontinued. Thus, corticosteroids are not used as a single agent for treating lymphoma. de Smet used a combination of MTX and dexamethasone in treating one patient with PCNSL-O resulting in complete remission. Castellino and associates reported the use of intravitreal corticosteroids injections with other systemic and intravitreal drugs [21]. However, intravitreal injections of corticosteroids did not become part of the standard practice in treating PCNSL-O.

Investigational Drugs for Intravitreal Injections

During the recent two decades, researchers reported their experience using various experimental drugs for intravitreal or intracameral injections in animal models of PCNSL-O. However, none of them has matured for clinical use.

Gregory and associates [59] studied the use of membrane FasL vesicles, the membrane-only form of Fas ligand, to activate innate immunity and terminate the eye's immune privilege. By a single injection of membrane FasL vesicles into the anterior chamber of mice, they eliminated the lymphoma cells that were previously injected into this site.

Li and associates [60] used recombinant immunotoxin HA22 targeting human B-cell lymphoma via their expression of CD22 in a mouse model of intraocular lymphoma. A single intravitreal injection of immunotoxin HA22 resulted in complete regression of the lymphoma, demonstrating B-cell-specific immunotoxin therapy.

Ublituximab is a glycoengineered anti-human-CD20 monoclonal antibody (similar to rituximab) developed to treat multiple sclerosis. In 2013 Ben-Abdelwahed and associates [61] reported their results in treating the murine model of PCNSL-O by a single intravitreal injection of ublituximab with marked effect against the lymphoma B-cells expressing CD20.

Some other monoclonal antibodies such as daclizumab, efalizumab, and alemtuzumab showed positive results in animal models and have the potential to be a useful adjuvant therapy for intraocular lymphoma [62]. However, as with previous experimental drugs, no further reports are available on their use in treating PCNSL-O.

Summary

Since intraocular lymphoma was first recognized about 70 years ago, its treatment has gradually evolved. Enucleation was often performed in the early years when the disease was diagnosed late. When PCNSL-O was more frequently diagnosed, and its common association with PCNSL-CNS was recognized, other methods of treatments have been used, including radiation therapy, systemic chemotherapy using various drugs, or in a combination of the two. The limited penetration of drugs administered systemically into the eye and their systemic toxicity, and the local side effects of radiation to the eye, paved the way for direct intravitreal chemotherapy to become the popular method of treating PCNSL-O in the last two decades.

Intravitreal injections of MTX as monotherapy were found to be very effective in inducing intraocular tumor remission with acceptable side effects and a rare occurrence of relapse when the entire 16 injections of the induction and consolidation phases are administered. Additional systemic chemotherapy probably neither adds to the cure rate of the PCNSL-O nor does it prevent PCNSL-CNS and should be used only when CNS lymphoma is associated with the PCNSL-O.

In recent years the use of intravitreal injections of rituximab has been carried out in several centers, with or without combining MTX, with encouraging results and no significant adverse effects. However, its use varies markedly among experts and the results are still inferior to MTX. Intravitreal injection of melphalan was also proved to be an effective drug, but at this time has been employed only in one ocular oncology center on a dozen patients.

Because of the rarity of PCNSL-O, international collaboration is needed for defining the role of intravitreal chemotherapy in eradicating this disease. The present drugs used clinically are effective, and probably a consensus on protocols for using them is needed. It seems that in the future, the treatment of PCNSL-O will continue to evolve, new drugs will be introduced, and new methods of intraocular delivery will be developed.

References

1. Habot-Wilner Z, Frenkel S, Pe'er J. Efficacy and safety of intravitreal methotrexate for vitreo-retinal lymphoma - 20 years of experience. Br J Haematol. 2021;194:92–100.
2. Coupland SE, Damato B. Understanding intraocular lymphomas. Clin Exp Ophthalmol. 2008;36:564–78.
3. Chaput F, Amer R, Baglivo E, Touitou V, Kozyreff A, Bron D, et al. Intraocular T-cell lymphoma: clinical presentation, diagnosis, treatment, and outcome. Ocul Immunol Inflamm. 2017;25:639–48.
4. Chan CC, Rubenstein JL, Coupland SE, Davis JL, Harbour JW, Johnston PB, et al. Primary vitreoretinal lymphoma: a report from an International Primary Central Nervous System Lymphoma Collaborative Group symposium. Oncologist. 2011;16:1589–99.
5. Kvopka M, Lake SR, Smith JR. Intraocular chemotherapy for vitreoretinal lymphoma: a review. Clin Exp Ophthalmol. 2020;48:240–8.
6. Hochberg FH, Miller DC. Primary central nervous system lymphoma. J Neurosurg. 1988;68:835–53.
7. Farrall AL, Smith JR. Eye involvement in primary central nervous system lymphoma. Surv Ophthalmol. 2020;65:548–61.
8. Pe'er J, Hochberg FH, Foster CS. Clinical review: treatment of vitreoretinal lymphoma. Ocul Immunol Inflamm. 2009;17:299–306.
9. Grimm SA, Pulido JS, Jahnke K, Schiff D, Hall AJ, Shenkier TN, et al. Primary intraocular lymphoma:

an International Primary Central Nervous System Lymphoma Collaborative Group Report. Ann Oncol. 2007;18:1851–5.
10. Kimura K, Usui Y, Goto H, Japanese Intraocular Lymphoma Study G. Clinical features and diagnostic significance of the intraocular fluid of 217 patients with intraocular lymphoma. Jpn J Ophthalmol. 2012;56:383–9.
11. Riemens A, Bromberg J, Touitou V, Sobolewska B, Missotten T, Baarsma S, et al. Treatment strategies in primary vitreoretinal lymphoma: a 17-center European collaborative study. JAMA Ophthalmol. 2015;133:191–7.
12. Coupland SE, Heimann H, Bechrakis NE. Primary intraocular lymphoma: a review of the clinical, histopathological and molecular biological features. Graefes Arch Clin Exp Ophthalmol. 2004;242:901–13.
13. Fend F, Ferreri AJ, Coupland SE. How we diagnose and treat vitreoretinal lymphoma. Br J Haematol. 2016;173:680–92.
14. Chan CC, Sen HN. Current concepts in diagnosing and managing primary vitreoretinal (intraocular) lymphoma. Discov Med. 2013;15:93–100.
15. Reichstein D. Primary vitreoretinal lymphoma: an update on pathogenesis, diagnosis and treatment. Curr Opin Ophthalmol. 2016;27:177–84.
16. Frenkel S, Pe'er J, Kaufman R, Maly B, Habot-Wilner Z. The importance of cytokines analysis in the diagnosis of vitreoretinal lymphoma. Acta Ophthalmol. 2020;98:e668–73.
17. Carbonell D, Mahajan S, Chee SP, Sobolewska B, Agrawal R, Bulow T, et al. Consensus recommendations for the diagnosis of vitreoretinal lymphoma. Ocul Immunol Inflamm. 2021;29:1–14.
18. Cooper EL, Riker JL. Malignant lymphoma of the uveal tract. Am J Ophthalmol. 1951;34:1153–8.
19. Vogel MH, Font RL, Zimmerman LE, Levine RA. Reticulum cell sarcoma of the retina and uvea. Report of six cases and review of the literature. Am J Ophthalmol. 1968;66:205–15.
20. Dalvin LA, Lim LS, Ancona-Lezama D, Mazloumi M, Chang M, Mashayekhi A, et al. Tumor control and visual acuity outcomes in vitreoretinal lymphoma with and without sub-retinal pigment epithelium infiltration: analysis of 125 eyes of 70 patients at a single ocular oncology center. Ophthalmol Retina. 2019;3:998–1005.
21. Castellino A, Pulido JS, Johnston PB, Ristow KM, Nora Bennani N, Inwards DJ, et al. Role of systemic high-dose methotrexate and combined approaches in the management of vitreoretinal lymphoma: a single center experience 1990-2018. Am J Hematol. 2019;94:291–8.
22. Cho BJ, Kim DY, Park UC, Lee JY, Yoon YH, Yu HG. Clinical features and treatment outcomes of vitreoretinal lymphoma according to its association with CNS lymphoma. Ocul Immunol Inflamm. 2018;26:365–71.
23. Yonese I, Takase H, Yoshimori M, Onozawa E, Tsuzura A, Miki T, et al. CD79B mutations in primary vitreoretinal lymphoma: diagnostic and prognostic potential. Eur J Haematol. 2019;102:191–6.
24. Ericson L, Karlberg B, Rosengren BH. Trials of intravitreal injections of chemotherapeutic agents in rabbits. Acta Ophthalmol. 1964;42:721–6.
25. Ericson LA, Rosengren BH. Present therapeutic resources in retinoblastoma. Acta Ophthalmol. 1961;39:569–76.
26. Seregard S, Kock E, Af Trampe E. Intravitreal chemotherapy for recurrent retinoblastoma in an only eye. Br J Ophthalmol. 1995;79:194–5.
27. Kaneko A. Teach us about the current treatments of retinoblastoma. Atarashii Ganka. 1996;13:229–33.
28. Kaneko A, Suzuki S. Eye-preservation treatment of retinoblastoma with vitreous seeding. Jpn J Clin Oncol. 2003;33:601–7.
29. Fishburne BC, Wilson DJ, Rosenbaum JT, Neuwelt EA. Intravitreal methotrexate as an adjunctive treatment of intraocular lymphoma. Arch Ophthalmol. 1997;115:1152–6.
30. Canellos GP, Lister TA, Skarin AT. Chemotherapy of the non-Hodgkin's lymphomas. Cancer. 1978;42:932–40.
31. de Smet MD, Vancs VS, Kohler D, Solomon D, Chan CC. Intravitreal chemotherapy for the treatment of recurrent intraocular lymphoma. Br J Ophthalmol. 1999;83:448–51.
32. de Smet MD. Management of non Hodgkin's intraocular lymphoma with intravitreal methotrexate. Bull Soc Ophtalmol. 2001:91–5.
33. Velez G, Yuan P, Sung C, Tansey G, Reed GF, Chan CC, et al. Pharmacokinetics and toxicity of intravitreal chemotherapy for primary intraocular lymphoma. Arch Ophthalmol. 2001;119:1518–24.
34. Smith JR, Rosenbaum JT, Wilson DJ, Doolittle ND, Siegal T, Neuwelt EA, et al. Role of intravitreal methotrexate in the management of primary central nervous system lymphoma with ocular involvement. Ophthalmology. 2002;109:1709–16.
35. Frenkel S, Hendler K, Siegal T, Shalom E, Pe'er J. Intravitreal methotrexate for treating vitreoretinal lymphoma: 10 years of experience. Br J Ophthalmol. 2008;92:383–8.
36. Sou R, Ohguro N, Maeda T, Saishin Y, Tano Y. Treatment of primary intraocular lymphoma with intravitreal methotrexate. Jpn J Ophthalmol. 2008;52:167–74.
37. Jeong Y, Ryu JS, Park UC, Oh JY. Corneal epithelial toxicity after intravitreal methotrexate injection for vitreoretinal lymphoma: clinical and in vitro studies. J Clin Med. 2020;9:2672.
38. Goldberg S, Frenkel S, Blumenthal EZ, Solomon A, Pe'er J. Intraocular lymphoma. Ophthalmology. 2007;114:1236–7.
39. Vicuna-Kojchen J, Frenkel S, Siegal T, Shalom E, Chowers I, Pe'er J. Maculopathy in patients with primary CNS lymphoma treated with chemotherapy in conjunction with blood-brain barrier disruption. Br J Ophthalmol. 2008;92:231–5.
40. Klimova A, Heissigerova J, Rihova E, Brichova M, Pytlik R, Spicka I, et al. Combined treatment

of primary vitreoretinal lymphomas significantly prolongs the time to first relapse. Br J Ophthalmol. 2018;102:1579–85.
41. Kaburaki T, Taoka K, Matsuda J, Yamashita H, Matsuda I, Tsuji H, et al. Combined intravitreal methotrexate and immunochemotherapy followed by reduced-dose whole-brain radiotherapy for newly diagnosed B-cell primary intraocular lymphoma. Br J Haematol. 2017;179:246–55.
42. Ma WL, Hou HA, Hsu YJ, Chen YK, Tang JL, Tsay W, et al. Clinical outcomes of primary intraocular lymphoma patients treated with front-line systemic high-dose methotrexate and intravitreal methotrexate injection. Ann Hematol. 2016;95:593–601.
43. Akiyama H, Takase H, Kubo F, Miki T, Yamamoto M, Tomita M, et al. High-dose methotrexate following intravitreal methotrexate administration in preventing central nervous system involvement of primary intraocular lymphoma. Cancer Sci. 2016;107:1458–64.
44. Abu Samra K, Oray M, Ebrahimiadib N, Lee S, Anesi S, Foster CS. Intraocular lymphoma: descriptive data of 26 patients including clinico-pathologic features, vitreous findings, and treatment outcomes. Ocul Immunol Inflamm. 2018;26:347–52.
45. Pulido JS, Johnston PB, Nowakowski GS, Castellino A, Raja H. The diagnosis and treatment of primary vitreoretinal lymphoma: a review. Int J Retina Vitreous. 2018;4:18.
46. Giuffre C, Cicinelli MV, Marchese A, Modorati GM, Brambati M, Ferreri AJM, et al. Clinical experience in a large cohort of patients with vitreoretinal lymphoma in a single center. Ocul Immunol Inflamm. 2021;29:472–8.
47. Kim H, Csaky KG, Chan CC, Bungay PM, Lutz RJ, Dedrick RL, et al. The pharmacokinetics of rituximab following an intravitreal injection. Exp Eye Res. 2006;82:760–6.
48. Pulido JS, Bakri SJ, Valyi-Nagy T, Shukla D. Rituximab penetrates full-thickness retina in contrast to tissue plasminogen activator control. Retina. 2007;27:1071–3.
49. Kitzmann AS, Pulido JS, Mohney BG, Baratz KH, Grube T, Marler RJ, et al. Intraocular use of rituximab. Eye (Lond). 2007;21:1524–7.
50. Mineo JF, Scheffer A, Karkoutly C, Nouvel L, Kerdraon O, Trauet J, et al. Using human CD20-transfected murine lymphomatous B cells to evaluate the efficacy of intravitreal and intracerebral rituximab injections in mice. Invest Ophthalmol Vis Sci. 2008;49:4738–45.
51. Ohguro N, Hashida N, Tano Y. Effect of intravitreous rituximab injections in patients with recurrent ocular lesions associated with central nervous system lymphoma. Arch Ophthalmol. 2008;126:1002–3.
52. Hashida N, Ohguro N, Nishida K. Efficacy and complications of intravitreal rituximab injection for treating primary vitreoretinal lymphoma. Transl Vis Sci Technol. 2012;1:1.
53. Larkin KL, Saboo US, Comer GM, Forooghian F, Mackensen F, Merrill P, et al. Use of intravitreal rituximab for treatment of vitreoretinal lymphoma. Br J Ophthalmol. 2014;98:99–103.
54. Cicinelli MV, Marchese A, Miserocchi E, Giuffre C, Berchicci L, Querques G, et al. Retinal and choroidal changes of vitreoretinal lymphoma from active to remission phase after intravitreal rituximab. Ocul Immunol Inflamm. 2020;28:637–46.
55. Fernandez Canabate E, Fernandez-Canabate S. [Intravitreal rituximab for the treatment of intraocular relapse of non-Hodgkin's lymphoma]. Farm Hosp. 2018;42:20–1.
56. Echegaray JJ, Llop S, Sepulveda M, Velez-Rosario R, Perez N, Oliver AL. Intravitreal rituximab for the treatment of a secondary intraocular relapse of a large B-cell lymphoma. Am J Ophthalmol Case Rep. 2018;9:77–9.
57. Shields CL, Sioufi K, Mashayekhi A, Shields JA. Intravitreal melphalan for treatment of primary vitreoretinal lymphoma: a new indication for an old drug. JAMA Ophthalmol. 2017;135:815–8.
58. Damato B, Bever GJ, Kim DJ, Afshar AR, Rubenstein JL. An audit of retinal lymphoma treatment at the University of California San Francisco. Eye (Lond). 2020;34:515–22.
59. Gregory MS, Koh S, Huang E, Saff RR, Marshak-Rothstein A, Mukai S, et al. A novel treatment for ocular tumors using membrane FasL vesicles to activate innate immunity and terminate immune privilege. Invest Ophthalmol Vis Sci. 2005;46:2495–502.
60. Li Z, Mahesh SP, Shen DF, Liu B, Siu WO, Hwang FS, et al. Eradication of tumor colonization and invasion by a B cell-specific immunotoxin in a murine model for human primary intraocular lymphoma. Cancer Res. 2006;66:10586–93.
61. Ben Abdelwahed R, Donnou S, Ouakrim H, Crozet L, Cosette J, Jacquet A, et al. Preclinical study of Ublituximab, a Glycoengineered anti-human CD20 antibody, in murine models of primary cerebral and intraocular B-cell lymphomas. Invest Ophthalmol Vis Sci. 2013;54:3657–65.
62. Rodrigues EB, Farah ME, Maia M, Penha FM, Regatieri C, Melo GB, et al. Therapeutic monoclonal antibodies in ophthalmology. Prog Retin Eye Res. 2009;28:117–44.

9 Ocular and Adnexal Lymphoma: Radiation Indications and Techniques

David Buchberger and Sheen Cherian

Introduction

Orbital lymphomas are uncommon, accounting for less than 1% of all lymphomas with an age adjusted overall incidence rate of 3.39 per million person-years [1, 2]. For the purpose of this chapter, ocular lymphoma can be classified into adnexal lymphoma (AL) and primary intraocular lymphoma (PIOL) [3]. The most common sites for AL are the bulbar conjunctiva, lacrimal gland, eyelid, and extraocular muscles [4]. PIOL mainly involves the uvea (choroid) or retina/vitreous.

Radiation Approach

Radiation dose and delivery techniques depend on the lymphoma location and specific histology. The orbit can be divided into three-thirds (anterior, mid, and posterior orbit) along its anteroposterior axis (Fig. 9.1) [5]. The anterior orbital lymphomas arise in the conjunctiva, eyelids, and nasolacrimal duct, while the mid orbital lymphomas arise in the extraconal space, intraconal space, extraocular muscles, lacrimal gland, and globe (uvea and retina/vitreous). The posterior orbital lymphomas are

D. Buchberger · S. Cherian (✉)
Department of Radiation Oncology, Cleveland Clinic, Cleveland, OH, USA
e-mail: BUCHBED2@ccf.org; cherias@ccf.org

V. R. Raval et al. (eds.), *Ocular and Adnexal Lymphoma*, Essentials in Ophthalmology,
https://doi.org/10.1007/978-3-031-24595-4_9

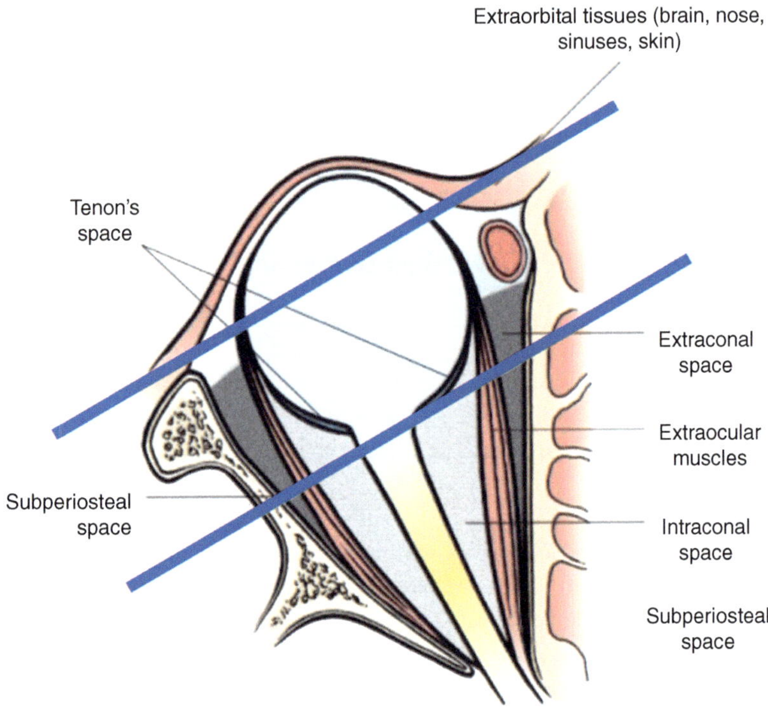

Fig. 9.1 Radiologic perspective: anatomy of the orbit

very rare, involving the orbital apex and the optic nerve. The critical structures for avoidance are cornea, lens, macula/fovea centralis, lacrimal gland, and optic nerve. Traditionally electron beam radiation therapy has been used for anterior orbital tumors and photon beam radiation therapy for mid and posterior orbital tumors.

Anterior Orbital Lymphoma

These tumors are typically anterior to the orbital septum and commonly involve the conjunctiva, nasolacrimal duct, and eyelids. They are mainly low-grade non-Hodgkin lymphoma (extranodal marginal zone lymphomas and follicular lymphoma).

Conjunctival and Nasolacrimal Duct Lymphoma

Best treated with an en-face electron field or photons using volumetric arc therapy (VMAT), as it allows sparing of the retina (macula) and optic nerve (Fig. 9.2a, b). Patients undergo contrast enhanced thin slice CT simulation, supine, eyes closed with a 3-point orfit mask for immobilization. Hard bolus is used on the orfit shell to pull away higher iso-dose lines (IDL) from the retina and optic nerve, and in the case of VMAT, its primary role is for dose buildup (prevent underdosing of conjunctiva/eyelid).

The clinical target volume (CTV) includes the entirety of the conjunctival sac (palpebral, forniceal, and bulbar conjunctival) together with gross tumor volume (GTV) or entire nasolacrimal duct together with GTV. A 2.5–3 mm isometric margin is added to CTV, creating the planning target volume (PTV). Recommended dose for low-grade NHL is 24 Gy/12 fx and 30 Gy/15 fx (consolidation radiation) for high-grade NHL. Approximately 15% of conjunctival lymphomas are bilateral at presentation; they are best treated with 3D conformal opposed lateral fields [3]. This allows better dose homogeneity without the need to match fields (Fig. 9.2c). Lens or cornea sparing is not advisable as this could lead to conjunctival underdosing and dose inhomogeneity. The risk of irreversible corneal damage is ≤5% at these doses, while cataracts from radiation are easily treated with cataract surgery.

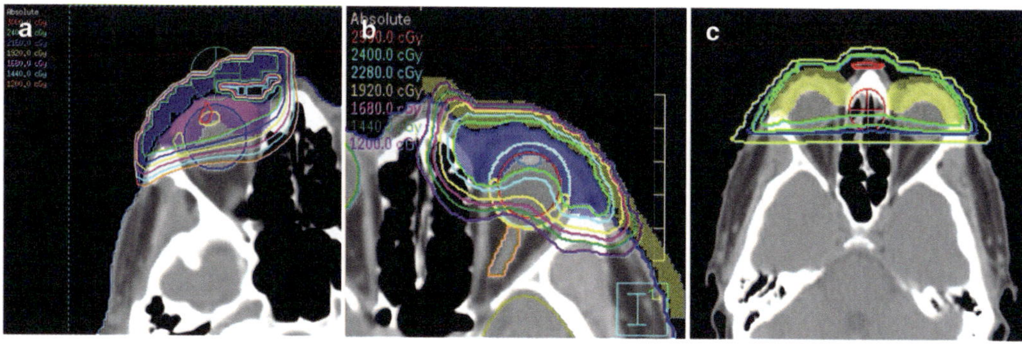

Fig. 9.2 Electron field treatment plan (**a**). VMAT radiation treatment plan (**b**). Opposed lateral photon beams used to treat bilateral conjunctival indolent lymphoma (**c**)

Eyelid Lymphoma

These are best treated with en-face electron beam and an eye shield. Clinical examination and high resolution axial imaging should confirm no disease extension beyond the orbital septum or involvement of bulbar conjunctiva. At simulation eyebrows are wired for sparing. Local anesthetic is instilled into the eye followed by placement of a soft contact lens to protect the cornea from abrasive effects of the eye shield. An appropriately sized eye shield is then placed on the eye and the eyelids are pulled over it and taped shut (Fig. 9.3a). A 3-point orfit mask is now utilized for immobilization. Next, a thin slice CT simulation is carried out. Automatic metal artifact reduction algorithms are utilized in the software setting to improve image quality. Hard bolus is used over the orfit mask during daily treatments, for dose homogeneity and buildup.

The GTV with an isometric margin of 3–5 mm restricted to the anterior aspect of the eye shield comprises the CTV, a further margin of 2.5–3 mm would create the PTV. In certain clinical situations when the GTV is not easily defined, the entire eyelid comprises the CTV (Fig. 9.3b, c). Final anterior posterior dimension of the PTV decides the energy of the electron beam.

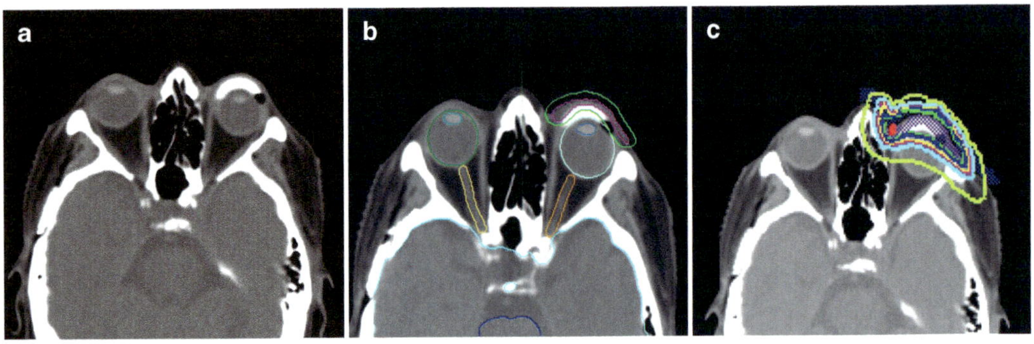

Fig. 9.3 Planning CT with eye shield in situ (**a**), showing CTV and PTV (**b**). Electron Beam plan with higher IDL sparing the cornea, lens, and retina (**c**)

Mid and Posterior Orbital Lymphoma

Mid and posterior orbital lymphomas are all treated with photons using VMAT radiation delivery techniques to spare the anterior elements of the orbit like the cornea, lens, and eyelids. These lymphomas have a predilection for the extraconal space, intraconal space, extraocular muscles, lacrimal gland, and globe (uveal tract and vitreous). Commonly seen tumors are diffuse large B-cell tumors and low-grade NHL of the lacrimal gland or extraocular muscles. They can also occasionally present as PIOL affecting either the retina/vitreous or uvea with no measurable disease activity elsewhere (CNS, CSF, or bone marrow).

In early stage, low-grade extranodal NHL, a definitive radiation dose of 24 Gy/12 fx is curative. In early stage, high-grade extranodal NHL, a course of systemic immuno-chemotherapy followed by consolidation radiation 30 Gy/15 fx is standard of care. In both instances of mid or posterior orbit lymphomas, the International Lymphoma Radiation Oncology Group (ILROG) recommends whole orbital radiation therapy as opposed to partial orbital radiation therapy, due to the higher incidence of local failure [3].

The process of radiation simulation is the same for AL affecting the mid or posterior orbit and PCNSL-O affecting the globe. Patients are scanned supine with IV contrast and a 3-point orfit mask for immobilization. In the case of PCNSL-O, 1 mm thickness, CT slices are recommended. Diagnostic image fusion to the planning CT scan might be needed for GTV delineation. For PCNSL-O affecting the retina/vitreous or uvea, the CTV includes the entire globe from ciliary body to the optic nerve up to the orbital apex. A 3–5 mm expansion on this CTV creates the PTV for treatment (Fig. 9.4a). In the case of AL the whole orbit becomes the CTV and a 3 mm isometric margin on the CTV creates the PTV (Fig. 9.4b–d).

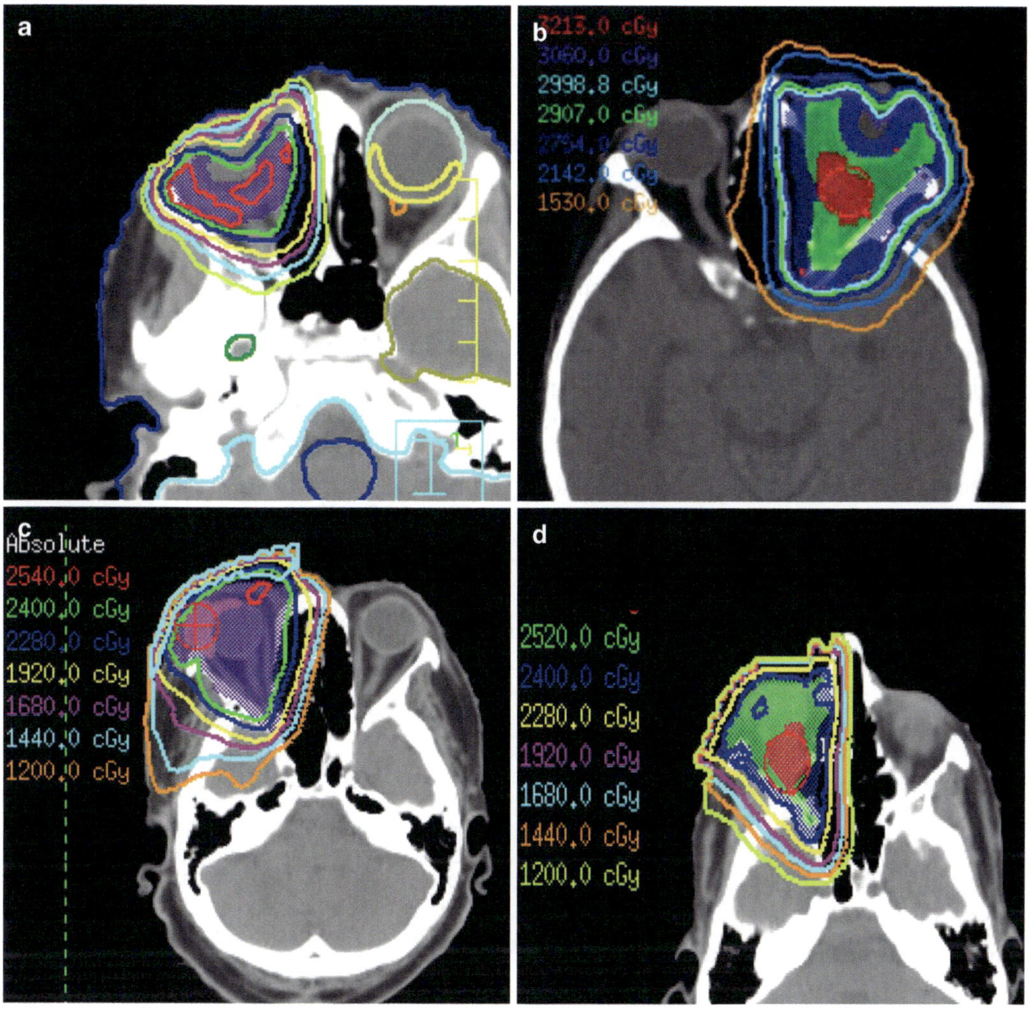

Fig. 9.4 Cornea and lens sparing VMAT for PCNSL-O (**a**); mid orbital AL (**b**), treated with lens sparing VMAT; lacrimal gland NHL treated with whole orbital RT (**c**); posterior orbital AL (**d**)

Indications, Efficacy, and Complications

Appropriate patient selection for external beam radiation therapy is pivotal. Prospective patients should be seen in a joint clinic with the ophthalmologist. Whenever possible staging investigations should precede tissue diagnosis, as this will avoid risks associated with orbital biopsies, as there could be an easily accessible extraocular site. Commonly used imaging modalities for AL are orbital MRI and PET/CT scan, while PCNSL-O is imaged using fundus photography, angiography (FA and ICG), autofluorescence, OCT, and ultrasonography (A-scan and B-scan) [6, 7]. Lymphoma blood work (CBC, BMP, LFT, ESR, and β2 microglobulin), bone marrow biopsy, CSF studies, and MRI brain are indicated for PCNSL-O.

Adnexal Lymphoma

Low-grade NHL (extranodal marginal zone and follicular lymphoma) are the commonest adnexal lymphoma seen in clinical practice. The ILROG recommends treating all stage IE ALs with external beam radiation therapy due to high-local control rates with low acute and late toxicity [3, 8]. Irrespective of location within the orbit, AL has an excellent prognosis, with local control and disease specific survival rates of 95% at around 5 years [9, 10]. Orbital radiation is well tolerated, requiring no treatment breaks. Transient acute side effects commonly seen are conjunctivitis, periorbital erythema, edema, excessive tearing, and mild pain. These symptoms almost completely resolve 4 weeks after radiation therapy. The major vision impacting long-term side effects with the exception of cataracts occur in less than 5% cases and they are radiation retinopathy, optic neuropathy, corneal erosion, dry eyes, and retinal hemorrhage [9, 10]. By using modern radiation techniques like VMAT, precise immobilization devices, eye shields, and daily image guidance, long-term toxicity can be kept to a bare minimum.

Primary Intraocular Lymphoma

High-grade NHL such as diffuse large B-cell lymphoma (DLBCL) is the commonest PCNSL-O encountered in clinical practice. Vitreo-retinal lymphoma is preferentially labeled as PCNSL-O to emphasize that it is an ocular variant or subset of primary CNS lymphoma (PCNSL). Those with concurrent CNS and ocular disease may be labeled as (PCNSL-CNS/O) in contrast to patients with CNS only involvement (PCNSL-CNS) at presentation. Diagnosis of PCNSL-O is made from vitrectomy, vitreous biopsy (vitreo/retinal lymphoma), or fine needle aspirate of choroid/uvea (uveal lymphoma) [11, 12]. Currently there is no standard of care guideline for treating PCNSL-O (vitreo/retinal lymphoma). Intravitreal methotrexate or ocular radiation therapy are acceptable options [13, 14]. Radiation alone results in approximately 60% local control and 94% overall survival rates at 2 years [12, 15]. However, response rates are more favorable for choroidal/uveal lymphoma [16]. Acute toxicities encountered commonly are tearing, conjunctivitis, dry eyes, orbital erythema, edema, loss of eyelashes, and mild orbital pain. Major vision impacting long-term side effects with the exception of cataracts occur in less than 5% cases and they are radiation retinopathy, optic neuropathy, dry eyes, retinal detachment, and retinal hemorrhage.

Conclusions

Modern radiation delivery techniques have vastly increased the precision and safety of orbital and globe radiation. This has resulted in significant reduction of radiation toxicity without compromising efficacy. Radiation continues to be a very efficient treatment modality for ocular and adnexal lymphomas.

References

1. Hassan WM, Bakry MS, Hassan HM, Alfaar AS. Incidence of orbital, conjunctival and lacrimal gland malignant tumors in USA from Surveillance, Epidemiology and End Results, 1973-2009. Int J Ophthalmol. 2016;9(12):1808–13.
2. Fitzpatrick PJ, Macko S. Lymphoreticular tumors of the orbit. Int J Radiat Oncol Biol Phys. 1984;10(3):333–40.
3. Yahalom J, Illidge T, Specht L, Hoppe RT, Li YX, Tsang R, et al. Modern radiation therapy for extranodal lymphomas: field and dose guidelines from the International Lymphoma Radiation Oncology Group. Int J Radiat Oncol Biol Phys. 2015;92(1):11–31.
4. Schwarcz RM, Coupland SE, Finger PT. Cancer of the orbit and adnexa. Am J Clin Oncol. 2013;36(2):197–205.
5. Cornelius CP, Mayer P, Ehrenfeld M, Metzger MC. The orbits--anatomical features in view of innovative surgical methods. Facial Plast Surg. 2014;30(5):487–508.
6. Aronow ME, Singh AD. The use of imaging in the diagnosis and management of intraocular lymphoma. Int Ophthalmol Clin. 2012;52(4):199–208.
7. Aronow ME, Portell CA, Rybicki LA, Sweetenham JW, Singh AD. Ocular adnexal lymphoma: assessment of a tumor-node-metastasis staging system. Ophthalmology. 2013;120(9):1915–9.
8. Portell CA, Aronow ME, Rybicki LA, Macklis R, Singh AD, Sweetenham JW. Clinical characteristics

of 95 patients with ocular adnexal and uveal lymphoma: treatment outcomes in extranodal marginal zone subtype. Clin Lymphoma Myeloma Leuk. 2014;14(3):203–10.
9. Platt S, Al Zahrani Y, Singh N, Hill B, Cherian S, Singh AD. Extranodal marginal zone lymphoma of ocular adnexa: outcomes following radiation therapy. Ocul Oncol Pathol. 2017;3(3):181–7.
10. Zhou P, Ng AK, Silver B, Li S, Hua L, Mauch PM. Radiation therapy for orbital lymphoma. Int J Radiat Oncol Biol Phys. 2005;63(3):866–71.
11. Stefanovic A, Davis J, Murray T, Markoe A, Lossos IS. Treatment of isolated primary intraocular lymphoma with high-dose methotrexate-based chemotherapy and binocular radiation therapy: a single-institution experience. Br J Haematol. 2010;151(1):103–6.
12. Teckie S, Yahalom J. Primary intraocular lymphoma: treatment outcomes with ocular radiation therapy alone. Leuk Lymphoma. 2014;55(4):795–801.
13. Raval V, Binkley E, Aronow ME, Valenzuela J, Peereboom DM, Wei W, et al. Primary central nervous system lymphoma: inter-compartmental progression. Eur J Haematol. 2022;3(2):362–70.
14. Raval V, Binkley E, Aronow ME, Valenzuela J, Peereboom DM, Singh AD. Primary central nervous system lymphoma - ocular variant: an interdisciplinary review on management. Surv Ophthalmol. 2021;66(6):1009–20.
15. Berenbom A, Davila RM, Lin HS, Harbour JW. Treatment outcomes for primary intraocular lymphoma: implications for external beam radiotherapy. Eye (Lond). 2007;21(9):1198–201.
16. Aronow ME, Portell CA, Sweetenham JW, Singh AD. Uveal lymphoma: clinical features, diagnostic studies, treatment selection, and outcomes. Ophthalmology. 2014;121(1):334–41.

Ocular Adnexal Lymphoma: Systemic Therapy and Clinical Trials

10

Allison Winter, Mary Aronow, Arun D. Singh, and Brian Hill

Introduction

Ocular adnexal lymphoma (OAL) is heterogeneous group of lymphomas, the majority of which are low-grade, indolent, B-cell, non-Hodgkin lymphomas (NHLs) [1]. OAL affects structures including the eyelids, conjunctiva, lacrimal apparatus, extraocular muscles, and sometimes the orbit. Disease may be limited to a single, localized tumor, or it may be multifocal. Overlap with ocular adnexal sites is common (10–20% of cases), and co-existing uveal involvement has been observed [2–6]. Moreover, OAL can affect regional, central, and peripheral lymph nodes as well as other distant extranodal sites. The 10-year, disease-specific mortality is approximately 5–10% [7]. Many of the advances in understanding OAL were initially demonstrated in systemic lymphoma (Box 10.1).

A. Winter · B. Hill (✉)
Taussig Cancer Institute, Cleveland Clinic, Cleveland, OH, USA
e-mail: wintera2@ccf.org; hillb2@ccf.org

M. Aronow
Retina Service, Department of Ophthalmology, Massachusetts Eye and Ear/Harvard Medical School, Boston, MA, USA
e-mail: mary_aronow@meei.harvard.edu

A. D. Singh
Cole Eye Institute, Cleveland Clinic, Cleveland, OH, USA
e-mail: singha@ccf.org

Box 10.1 Important Aspects of Ocular Adnexal Lymphoma (OAL)

- OAL consists primarily of five types of lymphoma, the most common of which is extranodal marginal zone type.
- The diagnosis depends on pathology, immunophenotypic analysis, and molecular genetics studies.
- Treatment of localized disease typically involves radiation therapy which results in excellent long-term local control.
- Systemic therapy with traditional chemotherapy or rituximab is reserved for aggressive histologic subtypes or those with systemic involvement.

Epidemiological Aspects

OAL is a rare disease, likely representing as many as 8% of all extranodal NHLs [1]. Its incidence is approximately 0.2 per 100,000 [8]. There is similar male and female predilection (60% of cases in most series) [9]. It affects most ethnic groups although there is significant geographic variation among systemic lymphoma, with the white population in the USA showing the highest incidence. The overall incidence of systemic OAL increases in a pattern which mirrors NHL [10].

V. R. Raval et al. (eds.), *Ocular and Adnexal Lymphoma*, Essentials in Ophthalmology,
https://doi.org/10.1007/978-3-031-24595-4_10

Among ophthalmic tumors, OAL comprises 6–8% of orbital and 10–15% of adnexal lesions [11–14]. Localized, ocular-only disease is present at diagnosis in 60–80% of cases, while the remainder have systemic involvement at the time of ophthalmic presentation [15, 16]. Bilateral disease is observed in 10–15% of individuals with ocular-only lymphoma [17]. Among affected ocular sites, the frequencies of involvement are conjunctiva 20–33%, orbit/lacrimal gland 46–74%, and eyelid 5–20% [7, 18]. Distinction between these sites can be difficult and combined involvement may be underreported [19, 20].

Many cases previously diagnosed as benign reactive lymphoid hyperplasia (BRLH) are now considered malignant lymphoma using current diagnostic techniques [21]. Retrospective studies of patients diagnosed with BRLH have revealed that up to 80% are now classified as malignant lymphoma [21]. At present, BRLH represents a minority of cases and is a diagnosis of exclusion.

Etiology and Pathogenesis: B-Cell Biology and Lymphomagenesis

The largest advances in understanding lymphoma pathogenesis and etiology as well as classification derive from the refined immunophenotypic [characterization of lymphocyte surface receptors, usually members of the clusters of differentiation (CD)] combined with concurrent advances in the understanding of molecular genetics of lymphocyte biology. This has resulted in a mechanistic hypothesis for lymphomagenesis which connects specific lymphoma types to different precursor cells and genetic events. Lymphoma classification, diagnosis, and pathogenesis are closely intertwined with their immunopathology and molecular biology.

The relationship between stages of lymphocyte development and their associated lymphoma diagnosis is based on distinct immunophenotypes. Tumors arise from germinal center cells (follicular lymphoma), cells of the mantle zone (mantle cell lymphoma), or memory B-cells (extranodal marginal zone lymphoma) all of which have undergone antigen exposure. From a molecular genetic standpoint, during normal lymphocyte maturation, somatic mutation may occur in which an antigen receptor gene region is juxtaposed to an oncogene region resulting in deregulation of the oncogenic region. Less often, a novel oncogenic protein is formed by fusion of two other genes. Chromosomal translocations underlying these alterations are well described in up to 90% of systemic lymphoma [22, 23]. Limited data suggests that these translocations are less common in OAL [24, 25].

The theory that lymphoma develops due to errors occurring during normal lymphocyte response to infection or inflammation is referred to as the infection/inflammation/mutation (IMM) model of lymphomagenesis. This has been corroborated in two ways. One is the recognized association of lymphoma with chronic antigen stimulation and infection, immune suppression, and autoimmune disease [26]. The prototypic example of the IMM model is gastric extranodal marginal zone lymphoma in which the endogenous mucosal-associated lymphoid tissue (MALT) develops lymphoma in response to chronic *H. pylori* infection. With the recent understanding that most OALs are also extranodal marginal zone lymphoma/MALT lymphomas, studies have shown evidence of DNA from infectious agents including *C. psittaci* and *H. pylori* in OAL [27, 28]. Infection as an underlying etiology for OAL shows variation among geographic regions and also within different series in the same geographic location [27, 29, 30]. Treatment implications of this are discussed below.

In addition to its therapeutic implications, perhaps the most important consequence of the IMM model is that it explains why the ocular adnexa, which has little if any endogenous lymphoid tissue, has lymphoma as its most common neoplasia. Similar mechanisms may occur in RLH. Based on the relative infrequency of OAL, there may be other factors required for lymphomagenesis.

Classification

OAL represents the malignant end of the spectrum of ocular adnexal lymphoproliferative disorders. As previously noted, BRLH and reactive lymphoid hyperplasia (RLH) with atypia represent a minority of cases and together comprise benign and intermediate forms of the disease, respectively [31, 32]. OAL is a localized form of lymphoma which has been integrated into the schema of lymphoproliferative diseases described in two major classification systems: the Revised European American Lymphoma classification in 1994 [33] and the 2008 World Health Organization (WHO) Classification of Tumors of Hematopoietic and Lymphoid Tissue [34].

OAL can be divided by the type and site(s) of tissue involvement. The vast majority of OAL are of the non-Hodgkin B-cell type. Despite the extensive numbers of systemic lymphoma subtypes, most OAL belong to one of the five subtypes: extranodal marginal zone (EMZL or MALT lymphoma), follicular lymphoma (FL), diffuse large B-cell lymphoma (DLBCL), mantle cell lymphoma (MCL), or lymphoplasmacytic lymphoma (LPL) (Table 10.1) [15, 20, 35–42]. The vast majority, approximately 80%, are of the EMZL type in most series [10].

OAL is termed solitary if it is the only site involved, secondary when contiguous sites are involved, and systemic if remote sites are involved. OAL is solitary in 60–80% of cases at the time of presentation [15, 35, 37, 42]. The rate of progression to systemic involvement can only be accurately identified using current criteria since misclassification was prevalent prior to the use of the WHO classification.

Table 10.1 Distribution of various types of ocular adnexal lymphoma

Author	Year	Patients	EMZL (%)	Follicular (%)	Mantle zone (%)	Lymphoplasmacytic (%)	Diffuse large B-Cell (%)	Plasmacytoma (%)	T-cell
White	1995	43	Not done						
Nakata	1999	44	77	–	4	2	14	–	–
Jenkins	2000	192	54	11	2	24	8		<1
McKelvie	2001	70	63	17	3		11		1
Shields	2001	117	Not done						
Mannami	2001	43	86	–	2	–	12	–	
Bhatia	2001	47	17	53			26		
Coupland	2003	230	59	12	3	4	13	4	3
Fung	2003	98	57	18	4		7		
Sharara	2003	17	47	12	18	6	18	–	
Cho	2003	57	98		2				
Sullivan	2005	69	35	22	1	4	7	3	6
Rosado	2006	62	89	–	–	–	<1	–	–
Ferry	2007	353	52	23	5	1	8	–	<1
Oh	2007	128	75	–	3	1	5	1	4
Hatef	2007	43	44	21	1	–	21	–	<1
Rootman	2011	122	60	12	1	4	4	–	–
Watkins	2011	57	28	2	5	–	4	4	5
Zanni	2012	41	63	10	5	5	17	–	–
Total		1833	17–98	11–53	1–18	4–24	1–26	1–4	1–6

Clinical Features

Symptoms

Subjective complaints in OAL are broad and may include: lacrimal gland, orbital, conjunctival mass or apparent eyelid mass, exophthalmos, pain, or diplopia. Many lesions are asymptomatic. If the lacrimal gland is involved, dry eye symptoms may occur.

Signs

OAL has site specific presentations which affect how the diagnosis is made. In the conjunctiva, lesions present typically with salmon or flesh pink color (Fig. 10.1). Clinical appearance does not allow distinction of benign from malignant lymphoproliferative disease. In the orbit, lacrimal gland, and eyelid, the lymphoma presents as a mass, which if palpable, is typically firm. Mobility is variable depending upon attachment to other structures. Diplopia may occur upon how rapidly the mass develops. Exophthalmos and decreased retropulsion of the globe may be the only clinical signs. Secondary ptosis may also occur (Fig. 10.2a). Involvement of the nasolacrimal drainage system can occur. Compression or invasion of the optic nerve can lead to vision loss. During orbital biopsy, OAL appears as a white to pink mass reflecting its leukocytic and vascular characteristics.

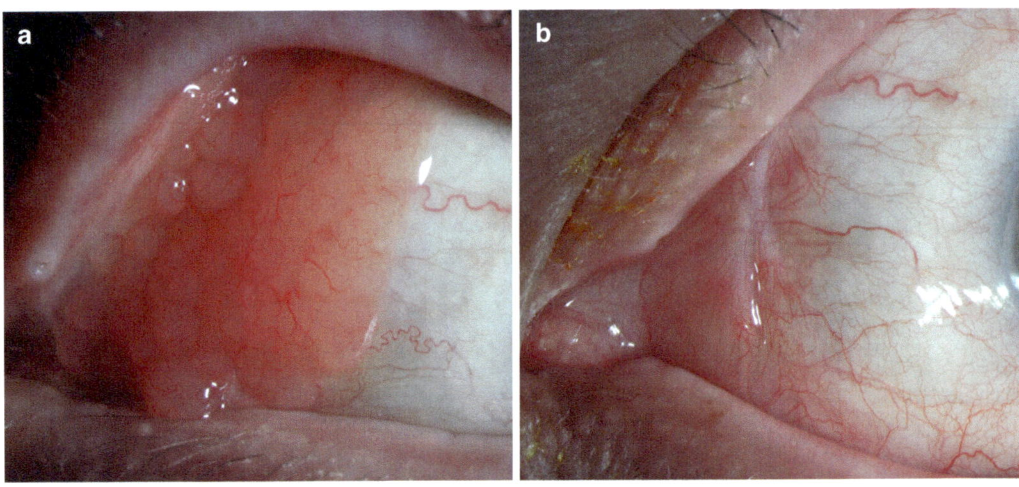

Fig. 10.1 Conjunctival lymphoma with typical salmon patch appearance (**a**). Note total regression following radiation therapy (24 Gy) (**b**)

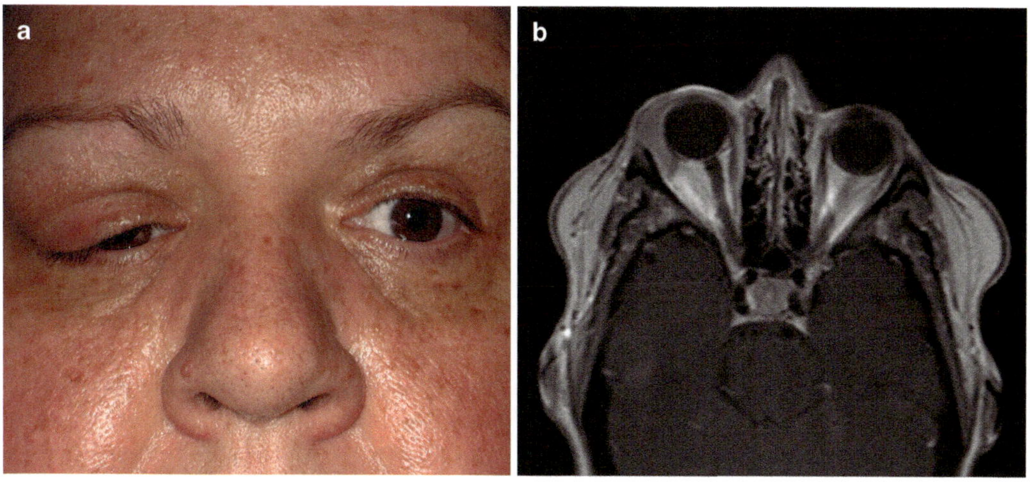

Fig. 10.2 Proptosis due to lymphoma involving the lacrimal gland (**a**). Coronal MRI scan (T-1 weighted image) demonstrating right orbital involvement (**b**). The infiltrating mass is in the existing normal anatomic spaces without distortion

Diagnostic Evaluation

Evaluation of OAL involves characterization of the lesion and staging. Biopsy should be obtained by open methods to allow sufficient material for multiple special studies: pathology, lymphocyte immunophenotypic analysis, and molecular genetic studies to identify gene rearrangements indicative of clonality and/or translocations.

Local Imaging Studies

Imaging studies of the orbit play an important role in OAL but are performed at different times depending on the presentation. With conjunctival disease, the lesion is frequently biopsied first and imaging of the orbit follows to assess orbital involvement. With orbital and lid disease, the orbit is usually imaged to optimize the biopsy process. Contrast enhanced CT and MRI scans of the orbits will show enhancing lesions which can be discrete or diffuse (Fig. 10.2b). Lymphoid lesions typically mold to structures such as the globe or bony orbit. Neuroimaging will reveal orbital lesions in up to 50% of clinically unsuspected cases [19]. Paranasal sinus involvement is not uncommon.

It is important to emphasize the frequency of overlap that occurs between OAL and uveal lymphoma [2–6]. For this reason, ancillary imaging studies such as B-scan ultrasonography and angiography are useful in characterizing the full extent and laterality of disease. This is particularly important in cases with subtle extrascleral extension (ESE) or occult involvement of the fellow eye. B-scan ultrasonography is a sensitive modality for detecting ESE. The pattern of ESE may be crescentic thickening, a discrete mass (often adjacent to the optic nerve), or diffuse choroidal thickening in cases where uveal lymphoma overlaps with OAL. Fluorescein (FA) and indocyanine green angiography (ICG) are also useful in suspected cases of uveal involvement. ICG demonstrates a characteristic pattern of focal hypofluorescence corresponding to clinically observed choroidal infiltrates. These foci may represent regions of choroidal nonperfusion secondary to space-occupying choroidal infiltration by lymphoma cells. ICG is superior to FA in visualizing the choroidal circulation and is therefore a particularly useful imaging modality in confirming the diagnosis and extent of disease burden [43]. When performed, FA may show early hyperfluorescence, hypofluorescent spots corresponding to clinically observed choroidal infiltrates, choroidal folds, or a normal angiogram.

Staging Procedures

Since OAL can co-exist with lymphoma in other sites, after OAL is classified, staging is performed. This includes a thorough physical examination by an experienced medical oncologist. Invasive staging has been replaced by the use of high resolution contrast enhanced imaging techniques: whole body PET/CDT or diagnostic CT of the chest, abdomen and pelvis, and MRI of the brain. Imaging of the neck is performed if cervical nodes are palpated or suspected to be enlarged. Laboratory evaluation includes complete blood count (CBC), hepatic enzymes, serum lactate dehydrogenase (LDH). Although part of the formal staging process for lymphoma, bone marrow aspiration, and biopsy has very low yield in patients with OAL. In the absence of cytopenias and radiographic evidence of systemic disease.

While not typically performed by the ophthalmologist, understanding the staging process is important for multidisciplinary management of OAL. The Ann Arbor staging system has several deficiencies for characterizing OAL, particularly as it results in a disproportionate staging distribution. Two-thirds of primary OAL cases present as a localized mass, which under the Ann Arbor system are classified as stage IE [15, 17, 44–48] (Table 10.2). Analysis can be challenging because of the use of different criteria but overall rates for initial staging are 60–80% for IE, 4–25% for IIE, and 16–18% for Stage III and IV combined [7, 36, 37]. Studies using criteria of extraorbital disease showed Stage III and IV rates of 22–36% at diagnosis [15, 35, 40]. This precludes the ability to differentiate the majority of OAL cases from one another based upon disease extent within the

Table 10.2 Staging of NHL by Ann Arbor and tumor-node-metastasis systems

Ann Arbor system	
Stage I	Localized or extranodal disease (Ann Arbor [AA] I or IE)
Stage II	2 or more nodal sites on same side of diaphragm
Stage III	2 or more nodal sites on both sides of diaphragm
Stage IV	Disseminated extranodal involvement (i.e. bone marrow, etc.)
B = B symptoms (unexplained fevers, drenching night sweats, or unintentional loss of >10% body weight)	
E = Extranodal involvement (visceral organ, ocular structures, skeletal lesions, etc.)	
Tumor-node-metastasis system[a]	
T Classification	TX Lymphoma extent not specified
	T0 No evidence of lymphoma
	T1 Conjunctival lymphoma alone
	T2 Orbital lymphoma with or without conjunctival involvement
	T3 Preseptal eyelid lymphoma in addition to conjunctival/orbital disease
	T4 Invasion of adjacent structures, such as bone and brain
N Classification	NX Lymph node involvement not assessed
	N0 No evidence of lymph node involvement
	N1 Involvement of ipsilateral regional lymph nodes
	N2 Involvement of contralateral or bilateral regional lymph nodes
	N3 Involvement of peripheral lymph nodes not draining ocular adnexal region
	N4 Involvement of central lymph nodes
M Classification	MX Lymphoma dissemination not assessed
	M0 No evidence of involvement of additional extranodal sites
	M1 Lymphoma involvement of other organs (at diagnosis or subsequently)

[a] Modified from the American Joint Committee on Cancer (AJCC) seventh edition TNM-based staging manual for OAL

ocular adnexal structures which may have important prognostic implications [18, 49].

More recently, a tumor-node-metastasis (TNM) based staging system for primary OAL has been developed under the guidance of the American Joint Committee on Cancer (AJCC) [50, 51]. (Table 10.2). This system addresses many of the shortcomings of the Ann Arbor system and more precisely defines disease extent. The ultimate goal of the proposed TNM-based system is to facilitate future studies aimed at identifying clinical and histopathologic features of OAL of prognostic significance and to assess treatment outcomes. To date, the feasibility of this system has only been analyzed in a limited capacity [52].

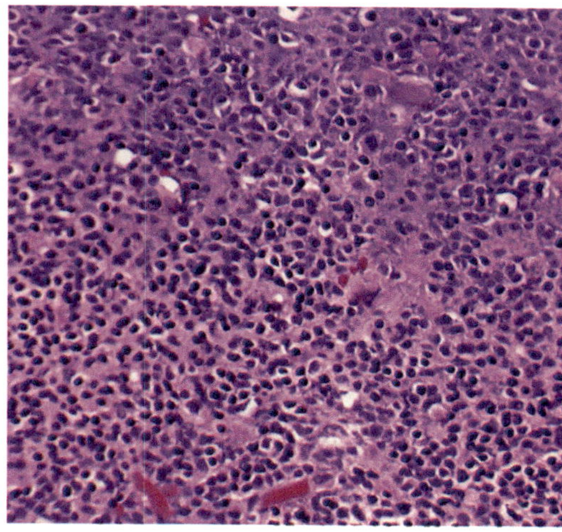

Fig. 10.3 Photomicrograph of monomorphic lymphocytes typical of EMZL type ocular adnexal lymphoma. (H&E, Original magnification × 100. Reproduced with permission from: Aronow ME, Hill BT, Singh AD. Orbital and adnexal lymphoma. Pe'er J, Singh AD (Editors) Clinical Ophthalmic Oncology. Volume 4, Chapter 15, Springer, Heidelberg (2019))

Differential Diagnosis

The clinical and imaging differential diagnosis of OAL is extensive, due to the paucity of specific features. It includes inflammatory lesions, benign lymphoproliferative lesions [32], epithelial tumors, melanocytic tumors, infectious lesions, and lacrimal gland lesions of the conjunctiva. In the orbit and lid, any mass including metastases, dacryoadenitis, inflammations, and other benign and malignant tumors must be considered.

Pathologic Features

Pathologic analysis can identify obvious lymphomas but cannot reliably differentiate lymphoma types (Fig. 10.3). Recent data has shown that using the current WHO classification, 76% of lesions previously classified as RLH are now reclassified as lymphomas. This is due to the recognition that a small number of malignant lymphocytes, whose presence is indicative of lymphoma, can be overshadowed by surrounding normal or reactive lymphoid cells. Immunohistochemistry can be carried out qualitatively on tissue sections or quantitatively on dispersed cells (flow cytometry). The use of intact tissue allows localization of marker expression, which can be critical in making the correct diagnosis. For example, overexpression of cytoplasmic Bcl-2 is not seen in normal follicular structures and is consistent with follicular lymphoma [32]. Immunohistochemistry, however, may not detect such critically important cells when sampling effect limits their presence. Flow cytometry, in contrast, does not give anatomic information but can accurately assign the immunophenotype of involved cells with very small amounts of specimen.

Molecular genetic analysis of OAL is important in two ways. Identification of overexpressed heavy chain gene rearrangements is indicative of clonality and typically represents malignancy. Tumor cells can be analyzed for translocations which may be indicative of a specific lymphoma type. Translocation of the MALT gene with API2 [t(11;18)(q21;q21)] is of specific interest since its presence is generally associated with more aggressive disease [53]. The expansion of the tools for lymphocyte characterization has paradoxically increased the chances for contradictory or incomplete characterizations using the new criteria. In such situations, the wisdom of an experienced hematopathologist is critical, though some lesions will remain unclassifiable.

Rare Variants

There are several rare variants and simulating conditions of OAL such as Langerhans cell histiocytosis (LCH), Rosai-Dorfman disease, T-cell lymphoma, T-cell/natural killer (NK)-cell lymphoma (lethal midline granuloma), and Burkitt lymphoma that we have included in this review.

Langerhans Cell Histiocytosis

LCH is characterized by a proliferation of Langerhans cells and inflammatory cells that generally affects children and young adults. The disease may be localized or it may affect multiple systems including the skin, bone, lungs, and lymphatics. Ophthalmic disease is observed in 10–23% of cases and most often manifests as a solitary lesion within the orbit; however, intraocular involvement in the form of an atrophic retinochoroidopathy has been reported [54–56]. Confirmation of diagnosis is made by biopsy, which demonstrates numerous histiocytes, giant cell formation, and eosinophilic granulocytes. Transmission electron microscopy (TEM) reveals characteristic intracytoplasmic Birbeck granules [55].

Rosai-Dorfman Syndrome

Also labeled as sinus histiocytosis with massive lymphadenopathy is a benign form of idiopathic histiocytosis that typically affects children and young adults. The majority of individuals (approximately 80%) develop painless cervical lymphadenopathy [57]. Extranodal involvement may affect multiple systems including the respiratory tract, skin, bones, visceral organs, and the central nervous system. The disease has multiple ophthalmic manifestations including lesions within the orbit, eyelid, and lacrimal apparatus. Compressive optic neuropathy, uveitic glaucoma, serous retinal detachment, and marginal corneal infiltrates have been reported [58]. Ocular adnexal involvement occurs in approximately 10% of patients with extranodal disease [59].

T-Cell Lymphoma

In rare cases, OAL can be of T-cell origin. In a review of 353 individuals with OAL, only a single case (0.3%) was of T-cell lineage [17]. As with B-cell neoplasms, a heterogeneous group of T-cell lymphomas can involve the ocular adnexal structures. Most T-cell lymphomas affecting the ocular adnexal structures are aggressive and carry a poor prognosis.

Most non-B-cell lymphomas are an extension of the malignant stage of mycosis fungoides or a secondary manifestation of systemic T-cell lymphoma. In a series of seven individuals with OAL of T-cell origin, three cases were peripheral T-cell lymphomas (PTCL) demonstrating positivity for CD3, CD8, and βF1 and negativity for CD56. Two cases were positive for CD3 and CD30 while negative for CD56 and were classified as anaplastic large-cell lymphomas of T-cell type (T-ALCL) [60]. The remaining two cases were positive for CD3 and CD56 and negative for βF1. These two cases were positive for Epstein-Barr virus (EBV) by in situ hybridization, consistent with T-cell/natural killer (NK)-cell lymphoma of nasal type (also referred to as lethal midline granuloma) [60, 61].

Burkitt Lymphoma

Burkitt lymphoma is a rare entity associated with translocation between chromosomes 8 and 14 affecting c-myc [62]. Three forms, all of which may affect the orbit, have been described. The African type frequently involves the orbits and maxillary bones and is associated with the presence of antibodies against Epstein-Barr virus (EBV) antigens [62]. The non-African type usually affects lymph nodes, bone marrow, and viscera. The third form affects immunocompromised individuals and is associated with acquired immunodeficiency syndrome (AIDS) [63–65]. Recent review of 16 immunocompetent individuals with sporadic orbital Burkitt lymphoma revealed a median age at diagnosis of 12 years [66]. Presenting symptoms included proptosis, ophthalmoplegia, and eyelid edema. Fourteen (88%) in this series had systemic involvement [66]. Biopsy of orbital lesions reveals a characteristic "starry-sky" appearance associated with Burkitt lymphoma [65]. Prognosis is guarded for this extremely aggressive lymphoma as significant mortality (54%) is observed within 1 year of presentation [66].

Treatment

The treatment of OAL is an area of controversy, progress, and change. Currently OAL treatment depends on whether the disease is localized or systemic. Local disease can be very effectively treated with radiation alone. Systemic disease is frequently treated in a manner similar to other indolent lymphomas, typically using rituximab alone or in combination with cytotoxic chemotherapy. With the recognition that the vast majority of OALs are of the EMZL/MALT type and that there may be an infectious basis for this subgroup of OAL, there is possibility of deferring cytotoxic modalities. A second controversy is whether to treat indolent OAL. A survey of treatment modalities follows.

Surgery

Surgery has been reported to be successful in managing certain cases of highly localized OAL and has been recommended for Stage I MALT systemic lymphoma in some sites. Its applicability remains dubious for most OAL due to the diffuse nature and frequent juxtaposition of OAL to sensitive ocular tissues. Surgery should therefore be reserved for localized, isolated lesions of the conjunctiva [7, 19].

Cryotherapy

Cryotherapeutic ablation of OAL has limited use in the management of OAL. It has resulted in variable success due to debulking the tumor without complete elimination of malignant tissue. It may have application in a limited number of patients with conjunctival OAL who are unable to receive other treatment modalities [20].

Radiation

Historically, external beam radiation (EBRT) has been the most frequently used modality for treatment of OAL. Analysis of this modality is confounded by small patient numbers in most series, the use of early and inaccurate classification schemes, short follow-up times, and apparent lack of ophthalmic follow-up. Complications were detected at a rate of up to 50% higher when close ophthalmic follow-up was performed.

Both electron and photon irradiation have been successfully employed in OAL. Dosage is based on the tumor grade or type [15, 35, 38]. Typical doses are 28–36 Gy for low-grade OAL and 30–40 Gy for high grade OAL. The role of lens shielding to decrease cataract formation is controversial with some studies showing no effect on local recurrence and others showing recurrences occurring in patients who underwent lens-sparing radiation treatment protocols [67, 68].

Analysis of radiation dose–response relationship of EMZL revealed that 5-year local tumor control rates of EMZL were 81% with doses below 30 Gy but 100% with doses higher than 30 Gy [69]. Variable sensitivity to radiotherapy based upon lymphoma subtype was observed as follicular lymphoma showed a 100% response rate to both high and low doses. While radiation studies frequently emphasize the ability to obtain local control, population-based observational data suggests that radiation may confer a survival benefit [70]. Even Stage IV-EA disease showed good local control, though survival was significantly lower. Multiple studies revealing higher rates of delayed systemic recurrence suggest that longer follow-up is necessary for accurate assessment of treatment effect [15].

Chemotherapy

Since OAL frequently presents as localized disease (stage IE), chemotherapy is rarely used, with the exception of aggressive DLBCL [71]. The review of chemotherapy used in lymphoma is beyond the scope of this chapter. Standard chemotherapy for OAL when it is part of more advanced disease is that of standard systemic lymphoma regimens using single agent rituximab alone or in combination with cyclophosphamide, doxorubicin, vincristine, and prednisone (CHOP), the alkylating agent chlorambucil and more recently, bendamustine which has dual properties of an alkylating agent and a purine analogue. While some have used systemic corticosteroids for tumor suppression of OAL, steroids offer ineffective long-term control.

Immunotherapy

Interferon

Interferon (IFN-alpha) has been used rarely for OAL despite its long standing use in systemic lymphoma. One report of five cases showed 80% initial complete response with short term follow-up [72]. One patient with Stage IIA disease died of systemic lymphoma at 1 year. More data regarding local and systemic efficacy are needed prior to acceptance of this modality.

Rituximab

Anti-lymphocyte antibodies are a recent form of lymphoma treatment. The most commonly used has been an antibody to CD20, rituximab, which leads to destruction of B-cells using mechanisms of complement and antibody mediated destruction as well as induction of apoptosis. These antibodies are effective when used alone but also significantly increase the remission rates when used in combination with chemotherapy [73].

Antimicrobial Treatment

A recent development in OAL management is based on the IMM model of lymphomagenesis. There is increasing evidence of the role of chronic infection in OAL. Both *C. psittaci* and *H. pylori* have been implicated [27, 28]. Follow-up data from *C. psittaci* detection studies have suggested a therapeutic effect following antibiotic therapy with doxycycline, presumably by eradication of the infection which underlies lymphomagenesis. Other studies have shown an effect in small numbers of patients using anti-*H. pylori* triple therapy [74]. Overall, antibiotic treatment regimens have shown variable results by study group and geographic location [30, 75]. Larger studies are needed to clarify the role of antibiotics in treatment of OAL.

Prognosis

Prognosis of OAL is evaluated in three ways: local control, systemic involvement, and death from lymphoma. Excellent local control has been reported using external beam radiation. Among OAL, EMZL has a quantitatively better prognosis than other tumor types with regard to spread of tumor and lymphoma related death, though the risk ratio was similar among the milder forms EMZL, LPCL, and FCL. The mortality ranges were: EMZL 0–20%, DLBCL 25–75%, FL 20–37%, MCL 38–100%, LPL 14–100% [7, 15, 35, 36].

Extraorbital spread can occur in over 45% of EMZL patients with mean follow-up of 63 months, suggesting that longer follow-up is needed [15]. Patients with indolent disease may survive decades without treatment.

Future Research

Future research will be focused on the mechanisms of lymphomagenesis to determine whether prelymphomatous conditions can be detected and treated with less toxic methods. One key question is whether the role of infectious agents will be as important as in gastric lymphoma where it has revolutionized care. Understanding lymphomagenesis may also allow for more targeted therapeutic agents.

References

1. Freeman C, Berg JW, Cutler SJ. Occurrence and prognosis of extranodal lymphomas. Cancer. 1972;29(1):252–60.
2. Fuller ML, Sweetenham J, Schoenfield L, Singh AD. Uveal lymphoma: a variant of ocular adnexal lymphoma. Leuk Lymphoma. 2008;49(12):2393–7.
3. Grossniklaus HE, Martin DF, Avery R, et al. Uveal lymphoid infiltration. Report of four cases and clinicopathologic review. Ophthalmology. 1998;105(7):1265–73.
4. Baryla J, Allen LH, Kwan K, Ong M, Sheidow T. Choroidal lymphoma with orbital and optic nerve extension: case and review of literature. Can J Ophthalmol. 2012;47(1):79–81.
5. Sarraf D, Jain A, Dubovy S, Kreiger A, Fong D, Paschal J. Mucosa-associated lymphoid tissue lymphoma with intraocular involvement. Retina. 2005;25(1):94–8.
6. Tagami M, Nagai T, Sekimukai D, Hara R, Azumi A. Uveal extranodal marginal zone B-cell lymphoma of the mucosa-associated lymphoid tissue type with concomitant extraocular lesions in a Japanese man. Jpn J Ophthalmol. 2011;55(5):585–7.
7. Coupland SE, Hellmich M, Auw-Haedrich C, Lee WR, Stein H. Prognostic value of cell-cycle markers in ocular adnexal lymphoma: an assessment of 230 cases. Graefes Arch Clin Exp Ophthalmol. 2004;242(2):130–45.
8. Cohen VM, Sweetenham J, Singh AD. Ocular adnexal lymphoma. What is the evidence for an infectious aetiology? Br J Ophthalmol. 2008;92(4):446–8.
9. Moslehi R, Coles FB, Schymura MJ. Descriptive epidemiology of ophthalmic and ocular adnexal non-Hodgkin's lymphoma. Expert Rev Ophthalmol. 2011;6(2):175–80.
10. Holm F, Mikkelsen LH, Kamper P, et al. Ocular adnexal lymphoma in Denmark: a nationwide study of 387 cases from 1980 to 2017. Br J Ophthalmol. 2021;105(7):914–20.
11. Shields JA, Bakewell B, Augsburger JJ, Flanagan JC. Classification and incidence of space-occupying lesions of the orbit. A survey of 645 biopsies. Arch Ophthalmol. 1984;102(11):1606–11.
12. Char DH. Orbital lymphoid lesions. Clinical Ocular Oncology. Philadelphia, PA: Lippincott-Raven; 1997. p. 349–64.
13. Henderson JW. The individual tumors orbital tumors. New York, NY: Raven Press; 1994. p. 44.
14. Spraul CW, Grossniklaus HE. Analysis of 24,444 surgical specimens accessioned over 55 years in an ophthalmic pathology laboratory. Int Ophthalmol. 1997;21(5):283–304.
15. Jenkins C, Rose GE, Bunce C, et al. Histological features of ocular adnexal lymphoma (REAL classification) and their association with patient morbidity and survival. Br J Ophthalmol. 2000;84(8):907–13.
16. Jenkins C, Rose GE, Bunce C, et al. Clinical features associated with survival of patients with lymphoma of the ocular adnexa. Eye (Lond). 2003;17(7):809–20.
17. Ferry JA, Fung CY, Zukerberg L, et al. Lymphoma of the ocular adnexa: a study of 353 cases. Am J Surg Pathol. 2007;31(2):170–84.
18. Knowles DM, Jakobiec FA, McNally L, Burke JS. Lymphoid hyperplasia and malignant lymphoma occurring in the ocular adnexa (orbit, conjunctiva, and eyelids): a prospective multiparametric analysis of 108 cases during 1977 to 1987. Hum Pathol. 1990;21(9):959–73.
19. Stafford SL, Kozelsky TF, Garrity JA, et al. Orbital lymphoma: radiotherapy outcome and complications. Radiother Oncol. 2001;59(2):139–44.
20. Shields CL, Shields JA, Carvalho C, Rundle P, Smith AF. Conjunctival lymphoid tumors: clinical analysis of 117 cases and relationship to systemic lymphoma. Ophthalmology. 2001;108(5):979–84.
21. Cockerham GC, Hidayat AA, Bijwaard KE, Sheng ZM. Re-evaluation of "reactive lymphoid hyperplasia of the uvea": an immunohistochemical and molecular analysis of 10 cases. Ophthalmology. 2000;107(1):151–8.
22. Ye H, Liu H, Attygalle A, et al. Variable frequencies of t(11;18)(q21;q21) in MALT lymphomas of different sites: significant association with CagA strains of H pylori in gastric MALT lymphoma. Blood. 2003;102(3):1012–8.
23. Raffeld M, Jaffe ES. bcl-1, t(11;14), and mantle cell-derived lymphomas. Blood. 1991;78(2):259–63.
24. Takada S, Yoshino T, Taniwaki M, et al. Involvement of the chromosomal translocation t(11;18) in some mucosa-associated lymphoid tissue lymphomas and diffuse large B-cell lymphomas of the ocular adnexa: evidence from multiplex reverse transcriptase-polymerase chain reaction and fluorescence in situ hybridization on using formalin-fixed, paraffin-embedded specimens. Mod Pathol. 2003;16(5):445–52.
25. Remstein ED, James CD, Kurtin PJ. Incidence and subtype specificity of API2-MALT1 fusion translocations in extranodal, nodal, and splenic marginal zone lymphomas. Am J Pathol. 2000;156(4):1183–8.
26. Hoover RN. Lymphoma risks in populations with altered immunity--a search for mechanism. Cancer Res. 1992;52(19 Suppl):5477s–8s.
27. Ferreri AJ, Guidoboni M, Ponzoni M, et al. Evidence for an association between Chlamydia psittaci and ocular adnexal lymphomas. J Natl Cancer Inst. 2004;96(8):586–94.
28. Chan CC, Smith JA, Shen DF, Ursea R, LeHoang P, Grossniklaus HE. Helicobacter pylori (H. pylori) molecular signature in conjunctival mucosa-associated lymphoid tissue (MALT) lymphoma. Histol Histopathol. 2004;19(4):1219–26.
29. Chanudet E, Zhou Y, Bacon CM, et al. Chlamydia psittaci is variably associated with ocular adnexal

MALT lymphoma in different geographical regions. J Pathol. 2006;209(3):344–51.
30. Husain A, Roberts D, Pro B, McLaughlin P, Esmaeli B. Meta-analyses of the association between Chlamydia psittaci and ocular adnexal lymphoma and the response of ocular adnexal lymphoma to antibiotics. Cancer. 2007;110(4):809–15.
31. Amin S, Ramsay A. Orbital and lacrimal gland progressive transformation of germinal centres--an underdiagnosed entity? Br J Ophthalmol. 2012;96(9):1242–5.
32. Stacy RC, Jakobiec FA, Schoenfield L, Singh AD. Unifocal and multifocal reactive lymphoid hyperplasia vs follicular lymphoma of the ocular adnexa. Am J Ophthalmol. 2010;150(3):412–26.e1.
33. Harris NL, Jaffe ES, Stein H, et al. A revised European-American classification of lymphoid neoplasms: a proposal from the International Lymphoma Study Group. Blood. 1994;84(5):1361–92.
34. Swerdlow S, Campo E, Harris NL, et al. Cancer TIAFRO. WHO classification of tumours of haematopoietic and lymphoid tissue (IARC WHO classification of tumours). 4th ed. Geneva: World Health Organization; 2008.
35. Fung CY, Tarbell NJ, Lucarelli MJ, et al. Ocular adnexal lymphoma: clinical behavior of distinct World Health Organization classification subtypes. Int J Radiat Oncol Biol Phys. 2003;57(5):1382–91.
36. McKelvie PA, McNab A, Francis IC, Fox R, O'Day J. Ocular adnexal lymphoproliferative disease: a series of 73 cases. Clin Exp Ophthalmol. 2001;29(6):387–93.
37. Mannami T, Yoshino T, Oshima K, et al. Clinical, histopathological, and immunogenetic analysis of ocular adnexal lymphoproliferative disorders: characterization of malt lymphoma and reactive lymphoid hyperplasia. Mod Pathol. 2001;14(7):641–9.
38. Bhatia S, Paulino AC, Buatti JM, Mayr NA, Wen BC. Curative radiotherapy for primary orbital lymphoma. Int J Radiat Oncol Biol Phys. 2002;54(3):818–23.
39. Sharara N, Holden JT, Wojno TH, Feinberg AS, Grossniklaus HE. Ocular adnexal lymphoid proliferations: clinical, histologic, flow cytometric, and molecular analysis of forty-three cases. Ophthalmology. 2003;110(6):1245–54.
40. Nakata M, Matsuno Y, Katsumata N, et al. Histology according to the Revised European-American Lymphoma Classification significantly predicts the prognosis of ocular adnexal lymphoma. Leuk Lymphoma. 1999;32(5–6):533–43.
41. White VA, Gascoyne RD, McNeil BK, Chang WY, Brewer LV, Rootman J. Histopathologic findings and frequency of clonality detected by the polymerase chain reaction in ocular adnexal lymphoproliferative lesions. Mod Pathol. 1996;9(11):1052–61.
42. Cho EY, Han JJ, Ree HJ, et al. Clinicopathologic analysis of ocular adnexal lymphomas: extranodal marginal zone b-cell lymphoma constitutes the vast majority of ocular lymphomas among Koreans and affects younger patients. Am J Hematol. 2003;73(2):87–96.
43. Saatci AO, Arikan G, Ozcan MA, Ozkal S, Kargi A, Undar B. Indocyanine green angiographic features of systemic non-Hodgkin's lymphoma and bilateral choroidal involvement. Ophthalmic Surg Lasers Imaging. 2006;37(3):236–9.
44. Coupland SE, Krause L, Delecluse HJ, et al. Lymphoproliferative lesions of the ocular adnexa. Analysis of 112 cases. Ophthalmology. 1998;105(8):1430–41.
45. Decaudin D, de Cremoux P, Vincent-Salomon A, Dendale R, Rouic LL. Ocular adnexal lymphoma: a review of clinicopathologic features and treatment options. Blood. 2006;108(5):1451–60.
46. Gardiner JA, White VA, Gascoyne RD, Rootman J. Histopathologic, immunophenotypic and genotypic analyses in ocular adnexal lymphoproliferative disorders. Aust N Z J Ophthalmol. 1992;20(3):247–51.
47. Hatef E, Roberts D, McLaughlin P, Pro B, Esmaeli B. Prevalence and nature of systemic involvement and stage at initial examination in patients with orbital and ocular adnexal lymphoma. Arch Ophthalmol. 2007;125(12):1663–7.
48. Plaisier MB, Sie-Go DM, Berendschot TT, Petersen EJ, Mourits MP. Ocular adnexal lymphoma classified using the WHO classification: not only histology and stage, but also gender is a predictor of outcome. Orbit. 2007;26(2):83–8.
49. Johnson TE, Tse DT, Byrne GE Jr, et al. Ocular-adnexal lymphoid tumors: a clinicopathologic and molecular genetic study of 77 patients. Ophthal Plast Reconstr Surg. 1999;15(3):171–9.
50. Coupland SE, White VA, Rootman J, Damato B, Finger PT. A TNM-based clinical staging system of ocular adnexal lymphomas. Arch Pathol Lab Med. 2009;133(8):1262–7.
51. AJCC. Cancer staging manual. 7th ed. New York, NY: Springer Science and Business Media LLC; 2009. www.springerlink.com. Accessed 18 Jan 2013.
52. Lee SE, Paik JS, Cho WK, et al. Feasibility of the TNM-based staging system of ocular adnexal extranodal marginal zone lymphoma of mucosa-associated lymphoid tissue (MALT lymphoma). Am J Hematol. 2011;86(3):262–6.
53. Liu H, Ye H, Dogan A, et al. T(11;18)(q21;q21) is associated with advanced mucosa-associated lymphoid tissue lymphoma that expresses nuclear BCL10. Blood. 2001;98(4):1182–7.
54. Moore AT, Pritchard J, Taylor DS. Histiocytosis X: an ophthalmological review. Br J Ophthalmol. 1985;69(1):7–14.
55. Herwig MC, Wojno T, Zhang Q, Grossniklaus HE. Langerhans cell histiocytosis of the orbit: five clinicopathologic cases and review of the literature. Surv Ophthalmol. 2012;58:330.

56. Thanos A, Vavvas D, Young LH, Foster CS. Choroidal neovascular membrane formation and retinochoroidopathy in a patient with systemic langerhans cell histiocytosis: a case report and review of the literature. Case Rep Ophthalmol. 2012;3(1):128–35.
57. Rosai J, Dorfman RF. Sinus histiocytosis with massive lymphadenopathy: a pseudolymphomatous benign disorder. Analysis of 34 cases. Cancer. 1972;30(5):1174–88.
58. Vemuganti GK, Naik MN, Honavar SG. Rosai Dorfman disease of the orbit. J Hematol Oncol. 2008;1:7.
59. Zimmerman LE, Hidayat AA, Grantham RL, et al. Atypical cases of sinus histiocytosis (Rosai-Dorfman disease) with ophthalmological manifestations. Trans Am Ophthalmol Soc. 1988;86:113–35.
60. Coupland SE, Foss HD, Assaf C, et al. T-cell and T/natural killer-cell lymphomas involving ocular and ocular adnexal tissues: a clinicopathologic, immunohistochemical, and molecular study of seven cases. Ophthalmology. 1999;106(11):2109–20.
61. Mendenhall WM, Olivier KR, Lynch JW Jr, Mendenhall NP. Lethal midline granuloma-nasal natural killer/T-cell lymphoma. Am J Clin Oncol. 2006;29(2):202–6.
62. Ruf IK, Rhyne PW, Yang H, et al. Epstein-Barr virus regulates c-MYC, apoptosis, and tumorigenicity in Burkitt lymphoma. Mol Cell Biol. 1999;19(3):1651–60.
63. Burkitt D. A sarcoma involving the jaws in African children. Br J Surg. 1958;46(197):218–23.
64. Reifler DM, Warzynski MJ, Blount WR, Graham DM, Mills KA. Orbital lymphoma associated with acquired immune deficiency syndrome (AIDS). Surv Ophthalmol. 1994;38(4):371–80.
65. Giuliari GP, Sadaka A, Cortez MA, Paniagua A. Orbital Burkitt's lymphoma: an aggressive presentation. Case Rep Ophthalmol Med. 2012;2012:354043.
66. Baker PS, Gold KG, Lane KA, Bilyk JR, Katowitz JA. Orbital Burkitt lymphoma in immunocompetent patients: a report of 3 cases and a review of the literature. Ophthal Plast Reconstr Surg. 2009;25(6):464–8.
67. Le QT, Eulau SM, George TI, et al. Primary radiotherapy for localized orbital MALT lymphoma. Int J Radiat Oncol Biol Phys. 2002;52(3):657–63.
68. Uno T, Isobe K, Shikama N, et al. Radiotherapy for extranodal, marginal zone, B-cell lymphoma of mucosa-associated lymphoid tissue originating in the ocular adnexa: a multiinstitutional, retrospective review of 50 patients. Cancer. 2003;98(4):865–71.
69. Platt S, Al Zahrani Y, Singh N, Hill B, Cherian S, Singh AD. Extranodal marginal zone lymphoma of ocular adnexa: outcomes following radiation therapy. Ocul Oncol Pathol. 2017;3(3):181–7.
70. Alderuccio JP, Florindez JA, Reis IM, Zhao W, Lossos IS. Treatments and outcomes in stage I extranodal marginal zone lymphoma in the United States. Cancers. 2021;13(8):1803.
71. Stacy RC, Jakobiec FA, Herwig MC, Schoenfield L, Singh A, Grossniklaus HE. Diffuse large B-cell lymphoma of the orbit: clinicopathologic, immunohistochemical, and prognostic features of 20 cases. Am J Ophthalmol. 2012;154(1):87–98 e1.
72. Blasi MA, Gherlinzoni F, Calvisi G, et al. Local chemotherapy with interferon-alpha for conjunctival mucosa-associated lymphoid tissue lymphoma: a preliminary report. Ophthalmology. 2001;108(3):559–62.
73. Sullivan TJ, Grimes D, Bunce I. Monoclonal antibody treatment of orbital lymphoma. Ophthal Plast Reconstr Surg. 2004;20(2):103–6.
74. Abramson DH, Rollins I, Coleman M. Periocular mucosa-associated lymphoid/low grade lymphomas: treatment with antibiotics. Am J Ophthalmol. 2005;140(4):729–30.
75. Ferreri AJ, Govi S, Pasini E, et al. Chlamydophila psittaci eradication with doxycycline as first-line targeted therapy for ocular adnexae lymphoma: final results of an international phase II trial. J Clin Oncol. 2012;30(24):2988–94.

Primary Central Nervous System Lymphoma: Neuro-Oncologic Approach

11

Ahmad N. Kassem and David M. Peereboom

Introduction

Primary central nervous system lymphoma (PCNSL) is defined as lymphoma confined to the central nervous system (CNS) at presentation. By contrast, secondary CNS lymphoma represents a systemic lymphoma (i.e., outside the CNS) that has metastasized to the CNS as a secondary site either as part of the initial presentation or at relapse. Conversely, up to 10% of patients with PCNSL develop systemic spread, typically late in the disease course [1].

PCNSL may involve the brain, eyes, leptomeninges, or the spinal cord. While ocular and adnexal lymphoma represents a subset of PCNSL, this chapter will address the management of PCNSL when it involves any of the remaining CNS compartments—i.e., the brain, leptomeninges, and the spinal cord. Spinal cord involvement is rare. PCNSL accounts for 2–3% of all primary CNS tumors [1]. The median age of patients with PCNSL is approximately 60 years. Over 90% of cases of PCNSL are classified histologically as diffuse large B-cell lymphoma (DLBCL) which is a particularly aggressive form of non-Hodgkin lymphoma (NHL) [2].

T-cell primary CNS lymphoma (TPCNSL) is a rare form of PCNSL and comprises 2–8.5% of cases, with higher incidences reported in eastern countries such as Japan and Korea [3]. The clinical picture and treatment modalities for T-cell PCNSL are similar to DLBCL with similar agents used in treatment, with the exception of rituximab, which is used only for B-cell malignancies.

Initial Diagnosis of CNS Lymphoma

About two-thirds of immunocompetent patients with PCNSL initially present with a solitary brain mass. Most patients present with focal neurological deficits and over 40% have neuropsychiatric symptoms. The brain hemispheres are most commonly involved (38%), followed by the thalamus and basal ganglia (16%), corpus callosum and related structures (14%), periventricular loci (12%), and the cerebellum (9%) [4]. MRI of the brain typically demonstrates periventricular homogeneous contrast enhancement with well-defined borders, low signal on T2-weighted imaging, and restricted diffusion on diffusion-weighted imaging (Fig. 11.1) [5]. Less typical presentations such as an intraventricular mass, cranial or radicular nerve enhancement, or isolated meningeal

The original version of the chapter has been revised. A correction to this chapter can be found at https://doi.org/10.1007/978-3-031-24595-4_12

A. M. Kassem
VCU Massey Cancer Center, Richmond, VA, USA

D. M. Peereboom (✉)
The Rose Ella Burkhardt Brain Tumor and Neuro-Oncology Center, Cleveland Clinic, Cleveland, OH, USA
e-mail: peerebd@ccf.org

V. R. Raval et al. (eds.), *Ocular and Adnexal Lymphoma*, Essentials in Ophthalmology,
https://doi.org/10.1007/978-3-031-24595-4_11

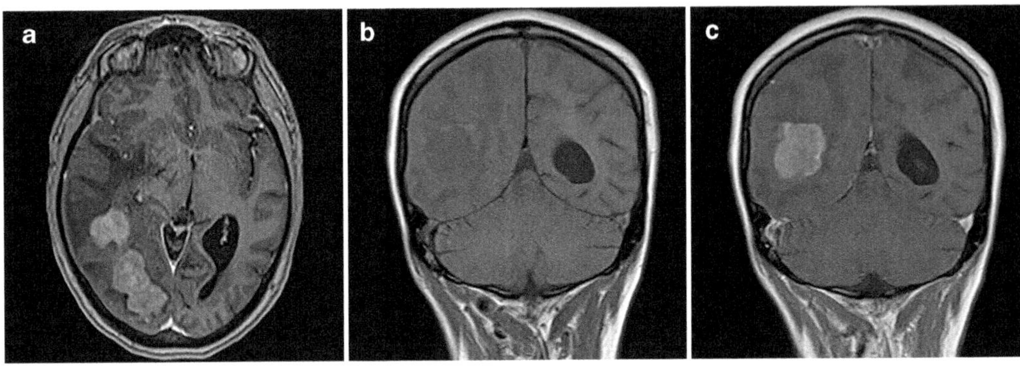

Fig. 11.1 There are multiple nearly confluent lesions in the right posterior parietal and occipital lobe (**a**, T1). Enhancement is present (**b**-before and **c**-after contrast injection)

enhancement have been described. Atypical imaging findings such as multiple ring-enhancing or patchy enhancing lesions can be seen in immunocompromised patients such as those with acquired immunodeficiency syndrome (AIDS) or post-organ transplant patients. Suggestive imaging must be followed by histopathologic confirmation. Tissue diagnosis is mandatory as the differential diagnosis on MRI of the brain includes multiple sclerosis, sarcoidosis, toxoplasmosis, and occasionally gliomas. Like lymphoma, these entities may demonstrate a transient response to corticosteroids [5]. Therefore, one must avoid corticosteroid administration prior to the proper evaluation of the patient with suspected PCNSL unless the patient is deteriorating. The potent lympholytic property of corticosteroids will commonly lead to necrosis of lymphoma, rendering tissue non-diagnostic.

Differentiating Primary and Secondary CNS Lymphoma

For a patient presenting with a possible CNS lymphoma on imaging, the initial decision on the site of tissue diagnosis depends on the presence or absence of other sites of disease; for this reason, imaging of the chest, abdomen, and pelvis typically with CT is necessary. Some centers use positron emission tomography (PET) CT scan with fluorodeoxyglucose (FDG) (PET-CT). Imaging allows one to distinguish primary from secondary CNS lymphoma; and in the case of the latter, to determine an alternative site for biopsy if suspicious imaging abnormalities exist. A lymph node is the biopsy site of choice, as it will reveal the lymph node architecture that informs the subtype of lymphoma and allows comprehensive molecular analysis, which in turn oftentimes will guide therapy. Men with negative systemic imaging should have a testicular ultrasound (US) to rule out primary testicular lymphoma, which, though uncommon as a primary site, has a significant risk of CNS metastasis [6]. If abnormal, a unilateral orchiectomy can be diagnostic. Bone marrow aspirate and biopsy have been recommended in some guidelines as part of the evaluation for systemic lymphoma. If imaging of the chest, abdomen, pelvis, and testis is negative, however, the likelihood of finding isolated bone marrow lymphoma as a source of CNS involvement is 2.5%, calling into question the utility of this procedure [7].

Once the CT of chest, abdomen, and pelvis and, in men, testicular US are confirmed negative, CNS tissue must be acquired to make a diagnosis. The following options should be pursued as needed, in order from least to most invasive.

1. Lumbar puncture (LP): If not contraindicated by elevated intracranial pressure, the least invasive method to diagnose PCNSL is an LP. Importantly, the CSF analysis should be of high volume (>10 mL) and must include flow cytometry and ideally review by a hematopathologist, in addition to routine analysis and cytology. CSF cultures are not necessary in the

absence of symptoms or signs of infection and omission of CSF cultures allows for prioritizing CSF to more relevant tests. Importantly, MRI should be performed *before* the LP to avoid nonspecific meningeal enhancement caused by the procedure. This enhancement can mimic leptomeningeal disease.

2. Slit lamp examination (SLE): SLE should be performed to detect cells in the vitreous and/or retinal infiltrates. A suspicious finding on SLE would be followed by a vitrectomy or, in some cases, by a retinal biopsy.
3. Brain biopsy: If both the LP and SLE are negative, the patient should have a brain biopsy. Although a positive LP or vitrectomy will spare the patient a brain biopsy, the patient who has been diagnosed by brain biopsy first should still undergo an LP and SLE to establish the presence or absence of disease in the CSF and/or ocular compartments, respectively. With a confirmatory brain biopsy, and suspicious findings on SLE, a vitrectomy is not needed. In case of a non-diagnostic biopsy after corticosteroid administration, serial imaging with MRI after withdrawal of corticosteroid therapy may be performed, typically at an interval of 6–8 weeks with repeat biopsy after radiologic evidence of tumor regrowth [8].

Prognosis and Goal of Treatment

The prognostic significance of the classic Ann Arbor staging system does not apply to PCNSL. Several prognostic scoring systems are used for PCNSL [9, 10]. The International Extranodal Lymphoma Study Group defines five parameters that correlated with a poor prognosis: age older than 60 years; performance status greater than 1 on the Eastern Cooperative Oncology Group performance status scale; elevated serum LDH; high CSF protein concentration; and tumor location within the deep regions of the brain (periventricular regions, basal ganglia, brainstem, and/or cerebellum). Patients with 0–1; 2–3; or 4–5 of these adverse risk factors had 2-year overall survival rates of 80%, 48%, or 15%, respectively [10]. The simplest prognostic score distinguishes three groups on the basis of age and Karnofsky performance status (KPS)—age <50 years; age >50 years and KPS >70; or age >50 years and KPS less than 70—which correlate with median overall survivals of 8.5 years, 3.2 years, and 1.1 years, respectively [9]. This system is easy to use in daily practice and offers a rough estimate of prognosis.

While age and performance status are important, several other details are taken into consideration. Organ dysfunction, comorbidity, and social support are factored in planning the treatment. A patient's suitability to receive high-dose chemotherapy and autologous stem cell rescue (HDC-ASCR) as part of initial therapy is one of the main management decisions in the treatment of PCNSL patients.

As with any serious illness, the optimal patient management is entry onto a clinical trial both at initial diagnosis and at disease progression. Unlike most CNS malignancies, the goal of therapy for PCNSL is long-term disease control. Most patients, even if severely ill, should be considered for aggressive treatment as PCNSL generally responds very well to therapy [11].

Immunocompetent Patient with PCNSL

PCNSL should be approached as a "whole-brain disease" [12]. Pretreatment clinical evaluation should include a detailed history and physical examination with careful assessment of neurologic deficits and lymphadenopathy, as the latter may suggest systemic disease. Cognitive function testing with neuropsychologic batteries should be performed at baseline if feasible, and during follow-up visits to monitor for potential treatment toxicities and to monitor cognitive function during and after treatment [13]. Patients at the time of diagnosis may be too ill to participate in such testing. Laboratory testing should include HIV and hepatitis serologies, lactate dehydrogenase, and hepatic and renal function tests.

There is no role for surgery in the therapeutic management of PCNSL. The rapid response to corticosteroids, chemotherapy, and radiation therapy obviates a role for surgical resection. On rare occasions, patients undergo surgical resection of a brain mass with radiological findings suggestive of a glioma, but for the pathology to reveal a lymphoma.

Before the advent of effective chemotherapy for PCNSL, whole-brain radiation therapy (WBRT) was the only treatment offered to PCNSL patients. WBRT resulted in short-lived responses with overall survival (OS) between 10 and 18 months with a 5-year survival of <20% [14, 15]. Furthermore, the neurocognitive decline seen in PCNSL survivors can be severe. Today, most centers defer WBRT until failure of effective chemotherapy regimens [16].

While WBRT is rarely used as part of initial therapy, stereotactic radiosurgery, the use of a highly conformal radiation plan for small lesions, can be used for the patient who has several small lesions. The definitions of "small" and "several" in this context vary with the particular institution but mean roughly less than 2 cm and fewer than 3–4 lesions, respectively. Several observational studies of SRS in PCNSL have been published [17].

The initial therapy for PCNSL is often considered according to three phases: induction, consolidation, and maintenance. Induction seeks to induce a complete response—the eradication of all of detectable disease. Consolidation is the use of subsequent therapy to eliminate remaining cancer to consolidate this response. Maintenance therapy strives to maintain this response by preventing recurrence of disease. While maintenance therapy is standard of care for the management of other hematological malignancies (e.g., acute leukemia), it is not uniformly considered standard for patients with PCNSL.

High-dose methotrexate (HD-MTX) is the most effective single agent in the treatment of PCNSL. Multiagent chemotherapy with a HD-MTX backbone is essential, yet the choice of agents to be used with MTX is still a matter of discussion [18, 19]. The addition of rituximab to MTX-based regimens has shown significant improvement in complete remission rates and OS. Rituximab, a standard of care for patients with systemic B-cell NHL, is part of nearly all induction protocols for PCNSL despite conflicting evidence as to its efficacy [20]. Multiple methotrexate-based chemotherapy regimens including rituximab have been investigated. Rituximab, methotrexate, vincristine, and procarbazine (R-MVP); rituximab, methotrexate, and temozolomide (MR-T); rituximab, methotrexate, etoposide, carmustine, and prednisone (RMBVP); and rituximab, methotrexate, cytarabine, and thiotepa (MATRix) are some of the commonly used induction regimens. The choice of induction regimen is largely determined by geographic tendencies and physician preferences as no regimen appears to be evidently superior [16]. The agents in the R-CHOP chemotherapy regimen (rituximab, cyclophosphamide, hydroxydaunorubicin (doxorubicin), Oncovin™ (vincristine), and prednisone), most commonly used in systemic lymphoma, have poor blood–brain barrier (BBB) penetration; this regimen thus has no role in PCNSL treatment.

Overall survival is the most important measure of efficacy of treatment for PCNSL. Radiographic response is assessed after induction and then after consolidation and with regular assessments after the completion of therapy. Radiographic responses are scored as complete response (CR), partial response, stable disease, and progressive disease (PD). The most important of these is the CR, which requires (1) complete disappearance of all enhancing abnormalities on contrast-enhanced MRI; (2) absence of malignant cells in the vitreous and resolution of any previously documented retinal or optic nerve infiltrates if present at initial staging; and (3) negative CSF cytology if previously positive [21].

Consolidation therapy is offered to patients who achieve complete or partial response after induction with the goal of achieving a durable response. Current consolidation therapy options include radiation, chemotherapy, or myeloablative chemotherapy with autologous stem cell rescue. Whereas some experts have retained WBRT as part of standard consolidation based on improved PFS, most have omitted WBRT based on the lack of OS advantage and the high rate of neurotoxicity with WBRT [22, 23]. More recent data, however, suggest the use of low dose (23.4 Gy rather than the typical 36–45 Gy) WBRT could have a role for consolidation therapy as evidenced by preliminary data that demonstrate efficacy with preserved neurocognitive status in patients who are not candidates for myeloablative chemotherapy with autologous stem cell rescue [24].

Patients with good organ function who achieve CR or near CR after induction therapy should be considered for consolidation therapy with high-dose chemotherapy and autologous stem cell rescue (HDC-ASCR). HDC-ASCR is commonly known as autologous bone marrow transplant. Patients should be carefully selected before undergoing such an aggressive treatment approach although the population eligible for HDC-ASCR is becoming more and more inclusive. Non-myeloablative consolidation with cytarabine and etoposide may be an attractive option to a wide population of patient who may not be eligible for HDC-ASCR [25].

The progress achieved in inducing and consolidating remission in PCNSL opened the door for discussion about maintenance therapy. Maintenance therapy uses less intensive therapy over a longer duration once a patient has achieved a CR (or in some cases a PR) with induction and consolidation therapy. One example is the use of obinutuzumab once every 2 months for 2 years currently being studied as a maintenance regimen (NCT02498951). Prospective studies are needed to confirm the benefit of maintenance therapy and to define the optimal agent. There is currently no consensus regarding a standardized follow-up for PCNSL patients. Patients should be reassessed after completion of therapy, at a minimum of every 3 months for 2 years, then every 6 months for 3 years, and annually for at least 5 years, for a total of 10 years of follow-up. Minimum testing at follow-up includes history, physical examination including a mini-mental status examination (MMSE), and gadolinium enhanced MRI scan of the brain. Ophthalmological follow-up intervals vary according to the patient's situation and should be coordinated with an ophthalmic oncologist.

Special Considerations for PCNSL in the Elderly

The incidence of PCNSL is increasing among the elderly, who comprise at least half of the individuals with this disease. Many PCNSL clinical trials exclude the elderly [18]. Elderly patients are at a higher risk of treatment toxicity due to declining organ function, decreased drug metabolism and elimination, comorbidities, and polypharmacy. The choice of induction therapy is particularly important in the elderly as they are often poor candidates for consolidation treatments. HD-MTX-based chemotherapy, however, is the treatment of choice for induction and is well tolerated by most elderly patients with adequate supportive measures and frequent checks of renal function [26]. Methotrexate and temozolomide; or methotrexate, vincristine, procarbazine, and cytarabine are potential induction regimens for elderly patients with PCNSL, with some studies slightly favoring the latter [27].

Immunosuppressed Patient with PCNSL

Immune suppression, either by HIV or immunosuppressive agents, allows growth of Epstein-Barr virus (EBV) which is known to drive lymphomagenesis. Immune suppression thus increases the risk of PCNSL and other NHL. The general strategy for management of these patients involves immune reconstitution—i.e., highly active antiretroviral therapy (HAART) in AIDS patients, or reduction of antirejection medicines in organ transplant patients—with or without cytotoxic therapy.

HIV-Associated PCNSL

PCNSL accounts for 15% of NHL in HIV patients versus less than 1% of NHL in the general population [28], with PCNSL constituting 30% of CNS lesions in patients with AIDS [29]. The frequency of HIV-associated PCNSL has diminished with the development of highly active antiretroviral therapy (HAART) [30]. Despite HAART, PCNSL has the worst prognosis of any HIV-associated malignancy, with an estimated 2-year mortality as high as 90% [31].

AIDS-related PCNSL (AR-PCNSL) typically occurs in patients with CD4 counts below 50 cells/μL blood [32]. Unlike the more insidious neurological decline seen in immunocompetent individuals, patients with AR-PCNSL often present with florid acute organic brain syndrome [28]. The diagnostic approach is similar to that in immunocompetent patients with a few differences. In addition to flow cytometry and cytology, CSF should be assayed for toxoplasma gondii and EBV. Detection of EBV activity in the CSF is suggestive of PCNSL. If CSF evaluation and ocular examination are negative and a brain biopsy cannot be performed, an elevated CSF EBV load in the setting of an FDG-avid CNS lesion on PET is highly specific and may justify treatment initiation [33].

AR-PCNSL is typically an end-stage manifestation of AIDS, and requires urgent immune reconstitution, to control both opportunistic infections as well as lymphoma. A challenge in AR-PCNSL is to effectively target the malignancy while allowing immune reconstitution.

Unfortunately, HIV seropositive individuals have been excluded from key studies in PCNSL treatment. Upfront WBRT with HAART had been considered the standard of care for AR-PCNSL but has largely been replaced by chemotherapy. HAART and HD-MTX should be considered as the first line for AR-PCNSL. Rituximab is safe in HIV-infected individuals and may be introduced when CD4 counts exceed 50 cells/μL [34]. Alkylating agents, vincristine and cytarabine, however, may be associated with an increased rate of neutropenic complications and a potentially more attenuated rate of CD4 recovery with HAART in HIV patients [32].

Iatrogenic Immunosuppression-Related PCNSL

The population of iatrogenically immunosuppressed individuals is steadily increasing with the wide use of immunosuppressive therapies and the advancements in the field of solid organ or allogeneic hematopoietic stem cell transplantation. Post-transplant lymphoproliferative disorder (PTLD) is a well-known complication of organ transplantation. Although brain involvement occurs in 7–15% of PTLD, isolated CNS disease is rare [35, 36]. For patients with PTLD, reduction of immunosuppressive drugs carries the risk of graft failure, which contributes to the high mortality [37]. Reduction of immunosuppression is therefore not adequate as a single strategy and must be accompanied by chemotherapy [35]. Close collaboration with the transplant providers is necessary in order to decide on how much to reduce the transplant antirejection regimen. The chemotherapy treatment regimens are similar to those used for immunocompetent patients.

Recurrent PCNSL

Despite the significant improvement in the management of PCNSL in the past years, up to 60% of patients experience relapse and one-third of patients have refractory disease (no response to initial therapy) [1, 38]. Treatment for progressive or refractory disease depends on performance status, site of relapse (e.g., brain parenchyma, CSF, and/or eyes), prior treatment, and duration of response [39]. In patients with long-lasting remission after initial treatment, re-challenge with a HD-MTX-containing chemotherapy should be considered [8, 40]. If HDC-ASCR was not attempted as a consolidation therapy, it may be offered upon relapse. Immunotherapy, inhibitors of Bruton tyrosine kinase such as ibrutinib, intrathecal rituximab, and other single agents or combinations may be considered [11].

After promising results in the treatment of secondary CNS lymphoma, CD19-directed chimeric antigen receptor (CAR) T-cells are in experimental use for the treatment of refractory or recurrent PCNSL. The treatment includes a lympho-depletion regimen prior to autologous CAR T-cell infusion [41]. The patients should be monitored for cytokine release syndrome, in addition to the typical complications of the conditioning regimen. Although the studies have included small numbers of patients, the results are promising.

Another option for salvage treatment of recurrent PCNSL or refractory is stereotactic radiosurgery (SRS). Used alone or with HD-MTX it should be considered in select patients. SRS appears to be more effective with small localized small lesions [42]. More prospective studies are needed to validate the efficiency of SRS in PCNSL. WBRT is also an option for patients with relapsed disease, generally reserved in situations where chemotherapy has become ineffective.

PCNSL with Leptomeningeal Involvement

Leptomeningeal dissemination occurs in up to 42% of patients with PCNSL [43]. Patients with leptomeningeal PCNSL may present with multifocal symptoms, headaches, cranial nerve palsies, and spinal radiculopathies; they often however present without localizing symptoms [44]. Primary leptomeningeal lymphoma (PLML) without synchronous parenchymal brain/spine or systemic disease is rare and constitutes about 7% of PCNSL cases [45].

In patients with obvious meningeal enhancement, intrathecal chemotherapy may have limited efficacy due to its very shallow penetration into the meninges. Nonetheless, current guidelines of the National Comprehensive Cancer Network (NCCN) recommend treatment with intrathecal MTX, cytarabine, or rituximab in cases of positive CSF studies or meningeal enhancement on MRI. Radiation therapy could be considered for the unusual patient in whom deficits and sites of disease are focal and chemotherapy by any route is not an option.

Diagnosis and Management of Neurological Complications of Treatment for PCNSL

Treatment-related neurotoxicity is defined as progressive neurological or cognitive impairment noted on serial examinations in the absence of lymphoma recurrence [46]. With the improvement in survival of patients with PCNSL, complications of treatment are more commonly observed and require significant attention.

WBRT alone or with systemic chemotherapy is a significant risk factor for the development of late neurotoxicity although lower dose WBRT regimens are being evaluated with the goal of avoiding this toxicity. Common symptoms and signs include deficits in attention, memory, executive function, gait ataxia, and incontinence. Patients over 60 years of age are at higher risk of developing treatment-related neurotoxicity. The MMSE is commonly used on follow-up to screen for this complication. The actual incidence of neurotoxicity may be underestimated as the MMSE has a low sensitivity for the detection of all of the symptoms of neurotoxicity.

Neurologic toxicity of HD-MTX can consist of stroke-like symptoms, an acute or subacute encephalopathy, and in the long term, a delayed multifocal leukoencephalopathy [47]. Rituximab uncommonly causes reactivation of John Cunningham (JC) virus leading to progressive multifocal leukoencephalopathy [48]. Vincristine neurotoxicity most commonly presents as a peripheral neuropathy. Cytarabine can cause an acute cerebellar ataxia. The prevention and management of iatrogenic neurotoxicity is an unmet need in the care of PCNSL patients and represents another role for the performance of clinical trials in the care of patients with PCNSL.

References

1. Jahnke K, et al. Relapse of primary central nervous system lymphoma: clinical features, outcome and prognostic factors. J Neuro-Oncol. 2006;80:159–65.
2. Phillips EH, Fox CP, Cwynarski K. Primary CNS lymphoma. Curr Hematol Malig Rep. 2014;9:243–53.
3. Bataille B, et al. Primary intracerebral malignant lymphoma: report of 248 cases. J Neurosurg. 2000;92:261–6.
4. Fine HA, Mayer RJ. Primary central nervous system lymphoma. Ann Intern Med. 1993;119:1093–104.
5. Küker W, et al. Primary central nervous system lymphomas (PCNSL): MRI features at presentation in 100 patients. J Neuro-Oncol. 2005;72:169–77.
6. Abrey LE, et al. Report of an international workshop to standardize baseline evaluation and response criteria for primary CNS lymphoma. J Clin Oncol. 2005;23:5034–43.
7. Hall KH, Panjic EH, Valla K, Flowers CR, Cohen JB. How to decide which DLBCL patients should receive CNS prophylaxis. Oncology. 2018;32:303–9.

8. Porter AB, et al. Primary central nervous system lymphoma can be histologically diagnosed after previous corticosteroid use: a pilot study to determine whether corticosteroids prevent the diagnosis of primary central nervous system lymphoma. Ann Neurol. 2008;63:662–7.
9. Abrey LE, et al. Primary central nervous system lymphoma: the memorial Sloan-Kettering Cancer Center prognostic model. J Clin Oncol. 2006;24:5711–5.
10. Ferreri AJM, et al. Prognostic scoring system for primary CNS lymphomas: the International Extranodal Lymphoma Study Group experience. J Clin Oncol. 2003;21:266–72.
11. Kassem AN, Peereboom DM. Approach to the patient with CNS lymphoma. Neuro-oncology for the clinical neurologist. Amsterdam: Elsevier; 2021. p. 172–85. https://doi.org/10.1016/B978-0-323-69494-0.00013-0.
12. Kerbauy MN, et al. Challenges and opportunities in primary CNS lymphoma: a systematic review. Radiother Oncol. 2017;122:352–61.
13. Grommes C, DeAngelis LM. Primary CNS lymphoma. J Clin Oncol. 2017;35:2410–8.
14. Shibamoto Y, et al. Results of radiation monotherapy for primary central nervous system lymphoma in the 1990s. Int J Radiat Oncol. 2005;62:809–13.
15. Nelson DF, et al. Non-Hodgkin's lymphoma of the brain: can high dose, large volume radiation therapy improve survival? Report on a prospective trial by the Radiation therapy Oncology Group (RTOG): RTOG 8315. Int J Radiat Oncol. 1992;23:9–17.
16. Citterio G, María Ferreri AJ, Reni M. Current uses of radiation therapy in patients with primary CNS lymphoma. Expert Rev Anticancer Ther. 2014;13:1327–37. https://doi.org/10.1586/14737140.2013.851007.
17. Alvarez-Pinzon AM, et al. Gamma knife stereotactic radiosurgery as an effective tool in primary CNS lymphoma: evaluation of stereotactic radiosurgery and methotrexate treatment in a prospective and observational clinical research study. Clin Neurol Neurosurg. 2021;201:106457.
18. Graham MS, DeAngelis LM. Improving outcomes in primary CNS lymphoma. Best Pract Res Clin Haematol. 2018;31:262–9.
19. Ferreri AJ, et al. High-dose cytarabine plus high-dose methotrexate versus high-dose methotrexate alone in patients with primary CNS lymphoma: a randomised phase 2 trial. Lancet. 2009;374:1512–20.
20. Bromberg JEC, van der Meulen M, Doorduijn JK. The role of rituximab in primary central nervous system lymphoma. Curr Oncol Rep. 2020;22:78.
21. Angelov L, et al. Blood-brain barrier disruption and intra-arterial methotrexate-based therapy for newly diagnosed primary CNS lymphoma: a multi-institutional experience. J Clin Oncol. 2009;27:3503–9.
22. Korfel A, Thiel E, Martus P, Weller M. Whole-brain radiotherapy in primary CNS lymphoma – authors' reply. Lancet Oncol. 2011;12:119–20.
23. Citterio G, Reni M, Gatta G, Ferreri AJM. Primary central nervous system lymphoma. Crit Rev Oncol Hematol. 2017;113:97–110.
24. Omuro AMP, et al. Randomized phase II study of rituximab, methotrexate (MTX), procarbazine, vincristine, and cytarabine (R-MPV-A) with and without low-dose whole-brain radiotherapy (LD-WBRT) for newly diagnosed primary CNS lymphoma (PCNSL). J Clin Oncol. 2020;38:2501. https://doi.org/10.1200/JCO.2020.38.15_suppl.2501.
25. Rubenstein JL, et al. Intensive chemotherapy and immunotherapy in patients with newly diagnosed primary CNS lymphoma: CALGB 50202 (Alliance 50202). J Clin Oncol. 2013;31:3061–8.
26. Bessell EM, Dickinson P, Dickinson S, Salmon J. Increasing age at diagnosis and worsening renal function in patients with primary central nervous system lymphoma. J Neuro-Oncol. 2011;104:191–3.
27. Neuwelt EA, et al. Primary CNS lymphoma treated with osmotic blood-brain barrier disruption: prolonged survival and preservation of cognitive function. J Clin Oncol. 1991;9:1580–90.
28. Rios A. HIV-related hematological malignancies: a concise review. Clin Lymphoma Myeloma Leuk. 2014;14:S96–S103.
29. Forsyth PA, DeAngelis LM. Biology and management of AIDS-associated primary CNS lymphomas. Hematol Oncol Clin North Am. 1996;10:1125–34.
30. Shiels MS, et al. Proportions of Kaposi sarcoma, selected non-Hodgkin lymphomas, and cervical cancer in the United States occurring in persons with AIDS, 1980-2007. JAMA. 2011;305:1450.
31. Achenbach CJ, et al. Mortality after cancer diagnosis in HIV-infected individuals treated with antiretroviral therapy. AIDS. 2011;25:691–700.
32. Gupta NK, et al. Long-term survival in AIDS-related primary central nervous system lymphoma. Neuro-Oncology. 2017;19:99–108.
33. Antinori A, et al. Value of combined approach with thallium-201 single-photon emission computed tomography and Epstein-Barr virus DNA polymerase chain reaction in CSF for the diagnosis of AIDS-related primary CNS lymphoma. J Clin Oncol. 1999;17:554.
34. Kaplan LD, et al. Rituximab does not improve clinical outcome in a randomized phase 3 trial of CHOP with or without rituximab in patients with HIV-associated non-Hodgkin lymphoma: AIDS-Malignancies Consortium Trial 010. Blood. 2005;106:1538.
35. Evens AM, et al. Primary CNS posttransplant lymphoproliferative disease (PTLD): an international report of 84 cases in the modern era. Am J Transplant. 2013;13:1512–22.
36. Morgans AK, Reshef R, Tsai DE. Posttransplant lymphoproliferative disorder following kidney transplant. Am J Kidney Dis. 2010;55:168–80.
37. Mahale P, Shiels MS, Lynch CF, Engels EA. Incidence and outcomes of primary central nervous system lymphoma in solid organ transplant recipients. Am J Transplant. 2018;18:453–61.

38. Langner-Lemercier S, et al. Primary CNS lymphoma at first relapse/progression: characteristics, management, and outcome of 256 patients from the French LOC network. Neuro-Oncology. 2016;18:1297–303.
39. Korfel A, et al. Randomized phase III study of whole-brain radiotherapy for primary CNS lymphoma. Neurology. 2015;84:1242–8.
40. Shenkier TN, et al. Primary CNS lymphoma of T-cell origin: a descriptive analysis from the international primary CNS Lymphoma Collaborative Group. J Clin Oncol. 2005;23:2233–9.
41. Siddiqi T, et al. CD19-directed CAR T-cell therapy for treatment of primary CNS lymphoma. Blood Adv. 2021;5:4059–63.
42. Palmer JD, et al. Outcomes after stereotactic radiosurgery for CNS lymphoma. J Neuro Oncol. 2020;147(2):465–76.
43. Korfel A, et al. Prognostic impact of meningeal dissemination in primary CNS lymphoma (PCNSL): experience from the G-PCNSL-SG1 trial. Ann Oncol. 2012;23:2374–80.
44. Taylor JW, et al. Primary leptomeningeal lymphoma: International Primary CNS Lymphoma Collaborative Group report. Neurology. 2013;81:1690.
45. Lachance DH, et al. Primary leptomeningeal lymphoma: report of 9 cases, diagnosis with immunocytochemical analysis, and review of the literature. Neurology. 1991;41:95–100.
46. Ferreri AJM, et al. Whole-brain radiotherapy in primary CNS lymphoma. Lancet Oncol. 2011;12:118–9.
47. Schaff LR, Grommes C. Updates on primary central nervous system lymphoma. Curr Oncol Rep. 2018;20:11.
48. Carson KR, et al. Progressive multifocal leukoencephalopathy after rituximab therapy in HIV-negative patients: a report of 57 cases from the Research on Adverse Drug Events and Reports project. Blood. 2009;113:4834.

Correction to: Primary Central Nervous System Lymphoma: Neuro-Oncologic Approach

Ahmad N. Kassem and David M. Peereboom

Correction to:
Chapter 11 in: V. R. Raval et al. (eds.), *Ocular and Adnexal Lymphoma*, Essentials in Ophthalmology, https://doi.org/10.1007/978-3-031-24595-4_11

Due to an unfortunate oversight, the name of Ahmad N. Kassem was inadvertently omitted as a co-author of Chapter 11. He has now been listed as the first author of this chapter. The necessary corrections have been made in both the Table of Contents and the chapter opener page to reflect the authorship.

The corrected authorship now reads as "Ahmad N. Kassem and David M. Peereboom", with the affiliations as follows:

Ahmad N. Kassem
VCU Massey Cancer Center, Richmond, VA, USA
E-mail: ahmadnkassem@gmail.com
David M. Peereboom
The Rose Ella Burkhardt Brain Tumor and Neuro-Oncology Center, Cleveland Clinic, Cleveland, OH, USA
E-mail: peerebd@ccf.org

The updated version of the chapter can be found at https://doi.org/10.1007/978-3-031-24595-4_11

V. R. Raval et al. (eds.), *Ocular and Adnexal Lymphoma*, Essentials in Ophthalmology,
https://doi.org/10.1007/978-3-031-24595-4_12

Index

V. R. Raval et al. (eds.), *Ocular and Adnexal Lymphoma*, Essentials in Ophthalmology,
https://doi.org/10.1007/978-3-031-24595-4

GPSR Compliance

The European Union's (EU) General Product Safety Regulation (GPSR) is a set of rules that requires consumer products to be safe and our obligations to ensure this.

If you have any concerns about our products, you can contact us on ProductSafety@springernature.com

In case Publisher is established outside the EU, the EU authorized representative is:

Springer Nature Customer Service Center GmbH
Europaplatz 3
69115 Heidelberg, Germany

Batch number: 10740038

Printed by Printforce, the Netherlands